MINOR SURGICAL PROCEDURES FOR

Nurses and Allied Healthcare Professionals

MINOR SURGICAL PROCEDURES FOR

Nurses and Allied Healthcare Professionals

Edited by
SHIRLEY MARTIN

John Wiley & Sons, Ltd

Other Wiley Editorial Offices

John Wiley & Sons Inc., 111 River Street, Hoboken, NJ 07030, USA
Jossey-Bass, 989 Market Street, San Francisco, CA 94103-1741, USA
Wiley-VCH Verlag GmbH, Boschstr. 12, D-69469 Weinheim, Germany
John Wiley & Sons Australia Ltd, 42 McDougall Street, Milton, Queensland 4064, Australia
John Wiley & Sons (Asia) Pte Ltd, 2 Clementi Loop #02-01, Jin Xing Distripark, Singapore
129809
John Wiley & Sons Canada Ltd, 6045 Freemont Blvd, Mississauga, ONT, L5R 4J3.

Wiley also publishes its books in a variety of electronic formats. Some content that appears in
print may not be available in electronic books.

Anniversary Logo Design: Richard J. Pacifico

Library of Congress Cataloging-in-Publication Data

Minor surgical procedures for nurses and allied healthcare professionals / edited by
  Shirley Martin.
    p. ; cm.
  Includes bibliographical references and index.
  ISBN-13: 978-0-470-01990-0 (pbk. : alk. paper)
  ISBN-10: 0-470-01990-5 (pbk. : alk. paper)
  1. Minor surgery.   2. Preoperative care.   3. Postoperative care.
  Martin, Shirley (Shirley Y.)
  [DNLM: 1. Surgical Procedures, Minor–methods.   2. Perioperative Care–
methods.   3. Preoperative Care–methods.   WO 192 M666 2007]
  RD111.M56 2007
  617'.024–dc22   2006030742

A catalogue record for this book is available from the British Library
ISBN 13: 978-0-470-0-1990-0

Typeset in 10/12pt Times by SNP Best-set Typesetter Ltd., Hong Kong
Printed and bound in Great Britain by TJ International Ltd, Padstow, Cornwall

This book is printed on acid-free paper responsibly manufactured from sustainable forestry in
which at least two trees are planted for each one used for paper production.

Contents

Part Three
Clinical Practices

List of Contributors

Rajesh Aggarwal, MA MRCS
Clinical Research Fellow, Department of Surgical Oncology & Technology, Imperial College, London

John Beesley, RGN LLM (Healthcare Law) BA (Hons)
Independent Perioperative Healthcare Consultant

Ann Clarridge, MSc BSc (Hons) Dip Th PGCEA RN DN
Principal Lecturer, London South Bank University

Verity Dansiger
Senior Solicitor, Capsticks, London

David Lomax, MBBS FRCA
Consultant Anaesthetist, St Mary's NHS Trust, London

Shirley Martin, RGN BSc (Hons)
Surgical Care Practitioner and Robotics Specialist Nurse, St Mary's NHS Trust, London

Christine McDougall RGN, Dip.Infection Control
Surveillance Manager, Surgical Site Infection Surveillance Service, Health Protection Agency

Debra Nestel BA PhD
Senior Lecturer in Communication, Department of Biosurgery and Surgical Technology, Imperial College, London

Barry Paraskeva PhD FRCS
Senior Lecturer and Consultant Surgeon, Imperial College and St Mary's Hospital, London

Anurag Patel BSc MRCS
Senior House Officer, ENT, Charing Cross Hospital, London

Sanjay Purkayastha
Clinical Research Fellow, Department of Surgical Oncology & Technology, Imperial College, London

Kausi Rao MBBS
Consultant Anaesthetist, Northwick Park Hospital, Harrow

Parvinderpal Sains MBChB MRCS
Specialist Registrar in General Surgery, Honorary Clinical Research Fellow, Imperial College and St Mary's Hospital, London

Julia Schofield MRCGP FRCP
Consultant Dermatologist, West Hertfordshire Hospitals NHS Trust

Jennifer Simpson RGN BSc (Hons)
Senior Surgical Care Practitioner, Department of Surgery, City Hospital, Birmingham

Gregory Thomas MBBS BSc
Senior House Officer in Surgery, St Mary's Hospital, London

Preface

This book is intended to provide nurses and allied healthcare professionals with the underlying theory, knowledge and skills they need to undertake minor surgical procedures. It is very much hoped that it will provide a helpful guide to those who have a specific interest in minor surgery.

Professor Sir Ara Darzi, KBE HonFREng FMedSci

Acknowledgements

The editor would like to thank the many contributors who willingly dedicated their busy time and committed to produce this book.

The editor would also like to extend her sincere thanks to Professor Sir Ara Darzi and the many other team members within the Academic Surgical Unit at Imperial College who gave support and encouragement which has helped to inspire the ideas presented in this book.

Finally I would like to thank my lovely family for their unwavering loyalty and continuing encouragement throughout this 'long winded' process.

Introduction

In recent years nursing has developed as a significant professional practice in its own right. This book has been written with the intention of providing nurses and allied healthcare professionals with a comprehensive guide that can be used as a reliable reference when performing minor surgical procedures. These encompass a range of benign and suspicious skin conditions which require simple surgical intervention.

This book will take the reader through a series of logical steps, highlighting significant issues and the principal limitations in practice. It has been primarily edited by an experienced practitioner with wide knowledge of the role of the non-medical practitioner in minor surgery. Various multidisciplinary professionals, including a consultant surgeon, anaesthetist, junior doctor, barrister, and an infection control nurse have contributed chapters, in addition to which assistance has been provided by many other experts.

Chapters within the book stand alone, enabling the reader to examine specific issues, for example the medico-legal implications involved in expanded roles for non-medical healthcare practitioners. The text is enhanced by illustrations, and a glossary is provided explaining the terminology used throughout.

Part One
Elementary Requirements

1 Starting Out: The Wider Picture

SHIRLEY MARTIN

Over the past decade the quality of differential care to patients has been transformed within the National Health Service (NHS) and primary healthcare settings. This process has led to the evolution of new roles for non-medically qualified practitioners working in a variety of specialist areas, and these new roles have created a myriad of clinical responsibilities. In addition, recent changes in medical manpower have resulted in the reduction of junior doctors' hours with specific shortages in many surgical specialties (The New Deal 1991; Calman 1993; Reilly et al. 1996; Working Time Directive 2004).

This chapter is intended to guide advanced specialist healthcare practitioners, such as Surgical Care Practitioners (SCPs) who are planning to undertake simple minor surgical procedures in a clinical setting. Whether the practitioner is considering the role for the first time or not, taking the first step may seem precarious; accompanied by many emotions, including apprehension and fear. This chapter will also focus on simplifying that transitional process, by acquainting practitioners with an overview of the many challenges likely to be faced, and will explore some of those simple but important questions which are likely to be encountered along the way.

Many practitioners today have been employed in senior roles comparable to that of a junior doctor and answerable to the consultant surgeon. However, many in this new field may not have perceived the hurdles that are likely to be encountered.

Firstly, it is essential that the practitioner questions how they might adjust to their transitional role and prepare for the many responsibilities that lie ahead. These questions should take place prior to, during and following the interview process. Subsequently it is important to look at how the role might be perceived and accepted by other medical trainees and patients, including nursing colleagues and multidisciplinary teams, as this could present many unexpected dilemmas, not considered prior to the appointment.

One of the most fundamental objectives is to highlight clearly how the practitioner will be clinically supported throughout their development, as this can be a long and tedious process involving many long hours of relentless work; which may often be accompanied by setbacks, and frustration. Strange

Minor Surgical Procedures for Nurses and Allied Healthcare Professionals. Edited by Shirley Martin.
© 2007 John Wiley & Sons Limited

as it may seem, these uncertainties arise time and time again. Unpublished reports suggest that many practitioners have yet to have their problems resolved even after a considerable amount of time spent in post.

Take a few minutes to examine the following questions.

- Will the practitioner use creativity to attain their goal?
- Will he or she survive the transition?
- Can he or she identify potential errors and thus improve potential for future achievements?

PRACTICAL STEPS TO LOCAL IMPLEMENTATION

- Consultant and management identify the specific needs of a training plan and clinical exposure within the organisation.
- Involve clinical governance to assure the quality of clinical services.
- Identify ongoing team development, clinical supervision, and mentorship by the clinician.
- Identify the employment strategy (Trust/Directorate).
- Identify where the practitioner is likely to be sited and establish if office space is available.
- Identify where the practitioner might obtain information technology (IT) as appropriate, to include Internet and Intranet access, to enable them to keep abreast of up to date information, including the latest relevant research.
- Consider how the practitioner might be contacted within the establishment's mobile phone/bleeps network.
- Ensure that the job title reflects the nature of the role.

These fundamental matters are integral to the first day if not first week of employment. It will not be surprising if some of these issues require many requisitions, endless paperwork and a variety of signatures.

THE PRACTITIONER

The practitioner may wonder why they have been appointed to their position. Only the employer can answer this question, There is no doubt that an individual who exudes enthusiasm will maintain the ability to think swiftly and make correct decisions, and it is essential that they demonstrate the ability to handle any stressful situations and rise to the challenges found along the way.

Practitioners must be made aware of the considerable groundwork required, and that this has to be undertaken on their own initiative. This will entail researching various aspects surrounding the role together with setting realistic goals. A worthwhile tip is to look at what has already been implemented before attempting to reinvent the wheel.

It is recommended that the practitioner starts with a little self-examination, and takes a few minutes to analyse the following.

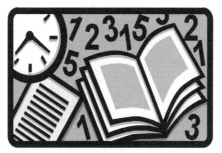

- Their own main strengths and weaknesses.
- Their overall ability, and capacity for making swift and judicious decisions when required.

Awareness in these areas will indicate the next steps to be taken, and where possible these should be discussed with the practitioner's supervisor as a part of self-assessment. The results of this exercise will lay the groundwork for the preparation of an individual development plan.

MULTI-TEAM SUPPORT

A collaborative form of approach of support, from a leading consultant surgeon, organisational managers, and the trust board is fundamental, to ensure that the role is developed to its full potential (Martin 2002).

It is also vital that the role is fully integrated, as this encourages cross-boundary multi-professional teamwork (Scholes and Vaughan 2002). This eliminates traditional boundaries, often regarded as the medial realm, allowing practitioners and doctors to work more closely. Organising meetings with others encourages a positive response and leads to a greater understanding of the additional support that may be required.

Such support includes secretarial and clerical support with access to referral letters and patient notes. Other areas such as ordering of diagnostic investigations plays a major part with the aspect of care and may entail the practitioner ordering pathological investigations and X-rays. It is essential that the practitioner's request is authorised. This will entail additional training and ratification at a local level.

Tips to consider are:

- do not appear over-confident or pretentious;
- remember to keep in touch with former colleagues;
- try not to work in isolation.

It is clear that the transition can present many potential pitfalls. The practitioner may initially encounter conflict and potential alienation from medical and nursing colleagues. Often mixed emotions surrounding the change can result in the practitioner working in isolation. There will inevitably be highs and lows and there may often be a need for 'a shoulder to cry on'. The question may arise as to whose shoulder might that be.

The following account demonstrates this well:

'The changes began the day I commenced my new role, which can only be described as one of the loneliest times of my life. There was excitement, but apprehension of the unknown was extremely daunting. The early days were crammed with introductions, meetings, visits and presentations; I was a novice in my own field of expertise. The doctors were very unsure of my role and I began to lose my own self-belief. My nursing colleagues treated me differently; and I felt as though I was no longer 'one of them'. How I missed the coffee room gossip and banter!

One of my problems was the unavailability of office space, and especially the lack of access to a personal computer. But as the days went by I grew more and more composed, my skills steadily developed and I began to engage confidently in previously unknown activities. The learning curve was steep but I have thrived in my new role and despite the early difficulties I realise now that this was the best step that I have ever made!'

SELF-MANAGEMENT?

It is important to understand that the practitioner may or may not be individually managed by more than one line manager/consultant. Self-management can often present a problem. For example, the line manager may believe that the management responsibility lies with the medical team, particularly if the practitioner is rostered as part of the surgical team. This often leads to unnecessary frustration over who is responsible for monitoring sickness, absence, annual leave, time owing and any other professional issues. Generally these issues should fall under the responsibility of the nurse/line manager. As a member of the extended surgical team the practitioner will be appointed on a day to day basis working under the direction of the consultant surgeon. Each practitioner is answerable to the consultant surgeon over the clinical management of the patient, but overall is responsible for their own activities and the management of their career.

Working alone may result in increased volume of work and heavier demands. It is therefore advisable that the practitioner devises a 'to do' duty list, to organise the urgent, important and not so important issues for each day. Sometimes additional tasks, such as preparing annual reports may have to be undertaken outside normal work hours.

JOB DESCRIPTION AND JOB TITLE

A job description should be formulated outlining the primary purpose of the new post and its essential functions. The duties listed in the job description must make clear the full extent of the knowledge, skills, and abilities necessary to perform the job. Any anticipated areas into which the role may develop should be incorporated as necessary. This is discussed in more detail in chapter 2.

Whilst many roles may have been locally initiated, misunderstanding and confusion over many differing job titles have become apparent. Titles such as Nurse Practitioner (NP), Clinical Nurse Specialist (CNS), Surgical Nurse Practitioner (SNP), Surgical Care Practitioner (SCP), and Perioperative Specialist Practitioner (PSP) are a few of the titles now being used.

As early as 1989, assistants in surgical practice within the operating department have been a part of the NHS as extended roles for nurses and operating department practitioners. Consultant surgeons in local trusts identified the need for the surgical assistant and developed the practitioner locally to meet service requirements, for example nurse-led carpal tunnel clinics and assisting in cardiac surgery. The role has subsequently expanded mostly in general surgery, cardiothoracic surgery and orthopaedics. In the operative phase, the surgical care practitioner can provide the same assistance to a surgeon as a trainee surgeon or perform an operative procedure delegated to them by the surgeon, for example, harvesting a vein or wound suturing.

In 2003 the title surgical practitioner was adapted by the National Association in Surgical Practice (NAASP). The working title of Surgical Care Practitioner was agreed after a Department of Health (2004) patient survey on titles was conducted. The patient survey identified an overall perception of the title Surgical Care Practitioner, the word 'care' was highlighted as it avoided the suggestion that the practitioner was a qualified doctor. Currently much debate continues, as it has been described as confusing and misleading (Moorthly et al. 2006). It is clear to state that the title first and foremost should be acceptable to patients indicating what the practitioners role is. Titles should be sufficiently distinct from titles already regulated and protected in law. This is discussed further in Chapter 2.

BUSINESS PLANNING

Strategic planning will enable the practitioner to identify and achieve any long-term goals of the service. The concept of formulating a business plan is to simplify those objectives by utilising a step by step guide, supported by evidence.

A business plan should include:

- the aim of the service to be provided;
- background of the role and the scope and boundaries involved;
- objectives and anticipated results;
- outcome measured in terms of time;
- financial and learning resources required, including information technology, personal IT equipment, and travel expenses for networking, courses and conferences;

- activities and hours involved in each, including following up results, correspondence and teaching commitments;
- administrative support;
- annual leave and essential cover;
- study leave to achieve the objectives of personal development plans;
- imminent but additional staff;
- review dates.

The practitioner may or may not have developed a business plan. If not it is well worth making the effort since it will provide a vision of where the future lies. All parties involved should develop this jointly. The importance of appropriate time planning will reap rewards.

CLINICAL GUIDANCE DOCUMENTS

The main purpose of clinical guidance documents is to standardise clinical practice to reflect the best available evidence, thus improving quality and equality. Clinical guidelines can help provide information and clarify best practice. It is essential that all members of the team are involved in preparing the relevant guidelines in order to to safeguard high standards of patient care. The process of ratifying written guidelines to permit practice may be slow within a practitioner's working environment, as it may be necessary for them to be approved by various steering committees or groups.

These are some of the issues considered by these bodies, taken from a report prepared in 1992 by the United Kingdom Central Council (UKCC):

- proposed adjustment to practice;
- proposed training, education and development programme;
- deemed competencies;
- clinical area applicable within the establishment;
- staff involved in development;
- staff with overall responsibility;
- development period: staff involved in approval;
- date approved;
- review date;
- presented to: (e.g. committee).

(List reproduced by kind permission of the Director of Nursing, St Mary's NHS Trust London)

Clinical guidance documentation may include:

- clinical history taking and examinations;
- requesting X-rays;
- performing interventional procedures (medical or surgical).

PROFESSIONAL INDEMNITY

It is apparent that variations exist among practitioners taking out additional professional indemnity for protection against consequences of negligence. It is advisable to explore this further, particularly when employed in the independent sector, as a number of employers insist on membership of an organisation such as the Medical Defence Union (MDU) or the Medical Protection Society (MPS). Although a majority of practitioners mainly work within the NHS it is worth while examining whether or not the government indemnity scheme is sufficient, and those is relying solely on this indemnity may find that they are unprotected. This is discussed in more detail in chapter 5.

Regulation

In 2005 the consensus for change outside nursing, the Shipman Inquiry and more so the scrutiny of the Doctor Regulator, led to an accompanying review of non-medical healthcare professional regulation, which was carried out on behalf of the Department of Health. The issue of regulating surgical care practitioners (SCPs) has been subjected to the Foster review (DH 2006b). There is currently discussion about a voluntary register of SCPs.

PERSONAL DEVELOPMENT ACTIVITY PLAN AND PORTFOLIO OF EVIDENCE

Compiling a personal development plan (PDP) provides an opportunity for the practitioner to identify short- and long-term objectives. Devising a PDP will contribute to any career aspirations. Essentially the practitioner's line manager should be the key person to help achieve the plan, completing a standard PDP form at the end of the process. The action plan should take into consideration:

- where the practitioner currently is and how the achievements have been accomplished;
- short- to long- term objectives;
- realistic goals;
- resources to support the practitioner;
- record of learning;
- further action necessary.

It is also essential that the practitioner be fully acquainted with plans to improve future services. Once the practitioner has established what the plans are, it may be necessary to develop a strategy for external developmental needs. These may include:

- enhancing communication skills – letter and report writing, skills for meetings and presentations;

- enhancing performance – organising own workload, communicating positively;
- development and improving research skills – writing research reports and material for publication;
- information technology – Word, Excel, Power Point, Access;
- Health & Safety – Advanced Life Support (ALS)/Intermediate Life Support (ILS) courses, manual handling, fire prevention and safety;
- leadership skills;
- accredited study courses/workshops, eg anatomy, history taking, prescribing;
- application for scholarships and awards;
- attend/shadow practitioners in similar roles in other institutions.

It is worth while registering with an established professional association relevant to practice, as this affords links with other practitioners and provides access to the latest developments, events, national issues and advancements applicable to practice.

The practitioner must be held responsible for upholding and reviewing their progress in ongoing knowledge and developments together with their experiences and competencies. Records of meetings with supervisors should be kept, together with notes of relevant topics discussed and key action points agreed. Any additional written plans should be referred to at each meeting and updated as appropriate.

PORTFOLIO OF EVIDENCE

A portfolio of evidence should include:

- clinical logbook;
- pre- and postoperative care (clinic/ward based areas);
- specific procedures performed;
- innovative developments, e.g. patient information leaflets;
- courses attended or participated in;
- record of visits and learning experiences;
- teaching involvement – nursing and medical staff;
- audit and research evaluation;
- competencies;
- reflective statements and personal experiences.

CLINICAL AUDIT

The Latin definition of audit encompasses the term 'to examine'. Clinical audit systematically reviews everyday care, and is widely used (NICE et al. 2002). It is undoubtedly an invaluable tool for improving quality care and clinical practice and should be acknowledged as an ongoing process rather than a one-off measure.

Clinical audit can evaluate:

- continuity of care;
- improved health outcomes;
- patient satisfaction;
- difference between health professionals;
- impact on services' waiting times, length of consultation, referrals;
- source of referral to the practitioner's clinic;
- patient and medical acceptability of advancing non-medical practitioner roles;
- managing risk assessment.

The audit cycle involves an observation of existing practice, the setting of standards, comparison between observed and set standards and the implementation of change.

Undertaking an audit to monitor and improve patient care can be rewarding and interesting rather then distressing and disheartening. Record keeping, however, can be tedious; therefore simple records/databases regarding the activity should for example identify the analysis of referrals and appointments, and in particular patient satisfaction surveys. In addition the audit should highlight how this data will be analysed and fed back. This may transform contemporary practices.

ANNUAL REPORT

Writing an annual report about the practitioner's role provides an excellent way of sharing their role with others within the organisation. It is essential that it identifies progress and achievements to date, and gives up to date information on patient/client groups, together with their needs and appropriate care.

The report should be clear, concise and well structured. Any data analysis should be included. Presentation of data should include a year-round picture rather than simply an end of year event. Effective and efficient data gathering and collation throughout the year will make this less time consuming as well as less stressful. The report should include:

- introduction;
- contents;
- the service;
- a review of the year;
- direct and indirect care;
- education and training;
- audit and research;
- future developments;
- summary and conclusion.

Reading relevant publications and annual reports will familiarise the practitioner with report writing styles. It may be worth while looking at the organisational website for additional guidance.

SPREADING THE WORD

Practitioners disseminating their work will have a positive impact upon the role being developed. It must be remembered that someone may be trying to establish a similar role elsewhere. Having the confidence to present at conferences locally and internationally is extremely rewarding. These events provide opportunities to meet external practitioners away from the organisation; they may also provide opportunities to sit on external board associations and steering groups relevant to the practitioner's work. Writing for publication is another way to share personal knowledge and interests. Selecting an appropriate subject, use a simple writing style which will attract the reader's attention. Reviewing books that have been recently published can be another way of entering the world of publication. Developing a relevant course enables practitioners to develop new and complex skills to take on new responsibilities. Entering into discussion with a university regarding a course developed by the practitioner for educational development towards a modular programme can lead towards a powerful course at an academically qualified level. It is fair to say that a high quality course will attract interest far and wide.

Organising an open day/evening can be advantageous, as this may provide the practitioner that one opportunity to meet and present their work to referring multidisciplinarians. Primary examples are referring healthcare professionals such as general practitioners and practice nurses. Such contacts foster opportunities to improve upon existing care.

POSITIVE OUTCOMES

Many factors can determine the success of the practitioner's role. One of the greatest rewards is gaining the support and gratitude of patients. It is essential that the practitioner takes time to pat themselves on the back, as such achievements make it all worth while. Earning respect and admiration from the surgical team can also be rewarding. Working to advance their knowledge provides the practitioner with greater job satisfaction and can embrace many targets set within governmental configurations.

SUMMARY

This chapter has introduced many of the key issues involved in developing a new role in clinical practice. These are exciting times for nursing and Allied

Health Practitioners. However there must be harmony and transparency between the role and its function. The practitioner should always remember that they are responsible for managing their own career. This requires self-belief, commitment and the ability to apply skills accordingly. Whilst a doctor traditionally performs the main role, it is fundamental that the essence of good practice is delivered throughout the whole episode of care. Both medical and management teams must wholeheartedly support these new practitioner roles and should recognise their full potential. The rest of the book explores a wide range of other matters surrounding role development and provides the reader with detailed guidance in many aspects of practice.

REFERENCES

Calman K (1993) Hospital doctors: training for the future. *Report of the Working Group on Specialist Medical Training*. London: Department of Health.

Department of Health (DH) (2006) *Optimising the Contribution of Non-Medical Healthcare Practitioners within Multi-Professional Teams – A Good Practice Checklist*. London: DH.

Department of Health (2006a) *The Curriculum Framework for the Surgical Care Practitioner*. National Practitioner Programme and the Department of Health. www.dh.gov.uk.

Department of Health (2006b) *Regulatrion of the Non-medical Health Professions*. London: DH. www.dh.gov.uk/assetRoot/04/13/72/95/04137295.pdf.

European Working Time Directive (2004) www.dh.gov.uk/assetRoot/04/08/26/35/04082635.pdf.

Martin S (2002) Developing the nurse practitioner's role in minor surgery. *Nursing Times* **98** (33), 39–40.

Medical Defence Union (MDU) www.the-mdu.com.

Medical Protection Society (MPS) www.mps.org.uk.

Moorthy R, Grainger J, Scott A, Powles JW, Lattis SG (2006) Surgical Care Practitioner – a confusing and misleading title. *Annals of the Royal College of Surgeons* (Suppl); **88**, 98–100.

National Association of Assistants in Surgical Practice (2005) *Surgical Care Practitioner*.

National Health Service Management Executive (1991) *Junior Doctors: The New Deal*. London: NHSME.

National Health Service Modernisation Agency (2004) *Public Perceptions of Surgical Practitioners*. London: NHSME.

National Institute for Clinical Excellence (NICE), Commission for Health Improvement (CHI) (2002) *Principles for Best Practice in Clinical Audit*. Oxford: Radcliffe Medical Press. www.nice.org.uk/pdf/BestPracticeClinicalAudit.pdf.

Reilly C, Challand A, Barrett A, Read S (1996) *Professional Roles in Anaesthetics: A Scoping Study*. Leeds: National Health Service.

Royal College of Surgeons *Surgical Care Practitioners* (in response to the front page article in the *Independent*, 6 December 2004).

Scholes J, Vaughan B (2002) Cross boundary working: implications for the multi-professonal team. *Journal of Clinical Nursing*; **11**, 399–408.
United Kingdom Central Council (1992) *The Scope of Professional Practice*. London: Nursing and Midwifery Council.

2 Modernisation: Role Redesign to Optimise Patient Outcomes

JOHN BEESLEY

The aim of this chapter is to outline the key social, professional and political drivers that have influenced the contemporary healthcare agenda. The chapter will outline the proliferation of new ways of working in medicine and surgery in response to these drivers and in particular how nurses and healthcare staff employed in professions allied to medicine are taking the opportunity to develop new career pathways. The chapter will outline how nurses and professions allied to medicine are embracing the modernisation agenda in response to national, local, service and patient needs.

The key political drivers that influence the contemporary modern healthcare agenda are:

- *NHS Plan: – a Plan for Investment, a Plan for Reform in England* (DH 2000a);
- Department of Health. *The NHS Improvement Plan: Putting People at the Heart of Public Services* (DH 2004);
- *Our National Health: a New Agenda in Scotland* (Scottish Executive 2000);
- *National Workforce Plan for NHS Scotland* (2004);
- *Improving Health: the NHS Plan for Wales* (Welsh Assembly 2001);
- *Developing Better Services: Modernising Hospitals and Reforming Structures in Northern Ireland* (2002).

In 1999 the introduction of devolution changed the nature of healthcare delivery within the United Kingdom (UK). Devolution was encouraged by the European Union (EU), the EU policy being to support the principle of subsidiarity, where decisions are taken as closely as possible to the people directly affected by the outcomes of those decisions. For example, the Welsh Assembly has moved decisions about issues such as healthcare from politicians at Westminster who may never have even lived in Wales to Welsh Assembly members in Cardiff, the home of the Welsh Assembly.

Devolution ensured that the national government of each home country controls healthcare spending and decides policy based on pertinent public

Minor Surgical Procedures for Nurses and Allied Healthcare Professionals. Edited by Shirley Martin.
© 2007 John Wiley & Sons Limited

service needs. Wales and Northern Ireland have their own Assemblies whilst Scotland has its own Parliament similar to England. There is a divergence of healthcare policy within the UK as a result of devolution. For instance, to date foundation Trust hospitals are only being set up in England.

Each home country has formulated and implemented its own individual healthcare plan in response to regional and local needs. The plans all have a common theme which is the overwhelming need to provide more investment in the NHS to ensure that it is fit to deliver a quality service to patients for the 21st century. The UK population is ageing, chronic illness is increasing and patients want more control and choice of services with less waiting and more familiar faces. This is the challenge healthcare providers face today. Reform is the key to modernisation of the NHS and this includes reviewing the way in which nurses and professions allied to medicine have traditionally administered care in the past.

NHS PLAN 2000

It is not in the scope of this chapter to outline all of the UK healthcare plans and their impact on modernisation and role redesign to optimise patient outcomes, but it is pertinent to concentrate on the NHS Plan in England which has resulted in a plethora of new ways of working in medicine and surgery.

The NHS Plan (England) is the most fundamental and far reaching reform programme in the history of the NHS. The vision of the plan is to deliver a health service designed around the needs of the patient. A key element of this transformation is new ways of working which will break down unnecessary boundaries between the professions, allowing healthcare staff to reach their full potential and improve services for patients. Old hierarchical ways of working are now giving way to support for the process of change, such as nurses training to be anaesthetic and surgical care practitioners, perioperative specialist practitioners and endoscopy practitioners. Public expectations with regard to prompt access to services are changing and so are professional roles. There is now more emphasis on a patient's needs and making better use of the expertise of non- medical practitioners. The NHS Plan identifies the need for a modern NHS workforce that works 'smarter not harder'.

The role of nurses, and all professionals within primary care, is being changed as a result of developments such as walk-in centres, NHS Direct, the treatment centre programme and GP surgeries undertaking more minor medical and surgical interventions.

The NHS Improvement Plan (DH 2004b) supports the commitment to a 10 year process of reform first set out in the NHS Plan 2000. Patients are receiving faster and more convenient access to care via improvements in GP services, accident and emergency waiting times, operations and treatment times. Many of the improvements have been made possible by NHS staff undergoing role redesign to be able to focus on the service needs of patients by reducing waiting times and offering a better service.

Everyone working within healthcare, regardless of occupational background or role has a duty to explore ways in which the quality of clinical services to the patient can be improved. This duty is integral to clinical governance and clinical effectiveness.

To promote and achieve a quality experience and positive outcome for patients requiring medical or surgical intervention the key core skills and competencies of all healthcare staff should be utilised. The staffing resource is therefore central to the quality assurance and modernisation agenda and proactive workforce development is crucial if healthcare organisations are to achieve the goals and vision of the NHS plans within the UK.

It is important to define what is innovative and new and what can be described as an extension of an established professional role. When setting up new roles it is essential that there is clarity about the job purpose and main functions of the role with the most important factor being whether the new role has a positive effect in the delivery of clinical services and patient outcomes. New roles have been introduced for a number of reasons, mainly the introduction and implementation of the European Working Time Regulations 1998 reducing the number of doctors' working hours, but also in response to personal interests and experience of individuals that have had the foresight to see how patient services can be improved by the addition of new skills. Those working in professions allied to medicine have responded with equal creativity to the modernisation agenda as have their nursing colleagues. Such innovative practice has been actively encouraged by the Department of Health with the formulation of career frameworks, namely the NHS Skills Escalator. The Skills Escalator is the structure by which the NHS will enable all levels of the workforce to acquire new skills and invest in professional development. Staff are encouraged through a strategy of lifelong learning to constantly renew and extend their skills and knowledge, thus giving them greater influence over their careers.

Many new clinical specialist roles are being created by nurses themselves who identify unmet patient needs. Nurses have a plethora of opportunities to progress their skills and knowledge while remaining in the frontline of patient care. Nurses can become specialists or even consultants in specialties such as wound care, stoma care, diabetes, continence, neonatal intensive care, pain management, palliative care, rheumatology and nutrition. In other areas non-medical practitioners are encouraged by medical colleagues to realise their potential and develop practitioner posts often supported by in-house competence based training to develop the necessary skills. The essence of this approach is that staff are encouraged through a strategy of lifelong learning to constantly renew and extend their skills and knowledge, enabling them to move up the skills escalator. Meanwhile, efficiencies and skill mix benefits are generated by delegating roles, work and responsibilities down the

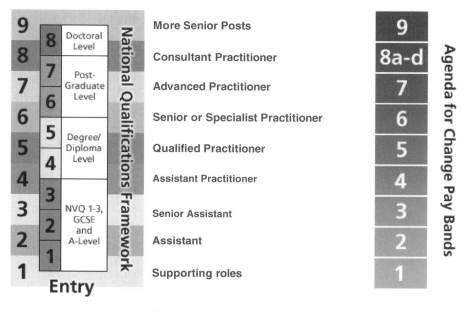

Figure 2.1 Career framework.

escalator where appropriate. Some staff may wish to develop their skills at a particular level of responsibility. Others may choose to develop the skills necessary for the next level of responsibility.

The Career Framework (CF), produced by Skills for Health, aims to provide a guide for NHS and partner organisations on the implementation of a flexible career and the Skills Escalator concept, enabling the individual with transferable, competency-based skills to progress in a direction which meets workforce, service and individual needs (figure 2.1).

CF level	CF Level Name	CF Level Description
1	Initial Entry Level Jobs	Jobs such as 'Domestics' or 'Cadets' requiring very little formal education or previous knowledge, skills or experience in delivering or supporting the delivery of healthcare.
2	Support Workers	Frequently with the job title 'Health Care Assistant' or 'Health Care Technician' – probably studying for or has attained NVQ Level 2.
3	Senior Healthcare Assistants/ Technicians	This is a higher level of responsibility than support worker, probably studying for or having attained NVQ Level 3, or Assessment of Prior Experiential Learning (APEL).

4	Assistant/Associate Practitioners	Probably studying for Foundation degree, BTEC higher or HND. Some of their remit will involve delivering protocol-based clinical care that had previously been in the remit of registered professionals, under the direction and supervision of a state registered practitioner.
5	Practitioners	Most frequently registered practitioners in their first and second post-registration/professional qualification jobs.
6	Senior/Specialist Practitioners	Staff having a higher degree of autonomy and responsibility than 'Practitioners' in the clinical environment; or who are managing one or more service areas in the non-clinical environment.
7	Advanced Practitioners	Experienced clinical professionals who have developed their skills and theoretical knowledge to a very high standard. They are empowered to make high-level clinical decisions and will often have their own caseload. Non-clinical staff at Level 7 will typically be managing a number of service areas.
8	Consultant Practitioners	Staff working at a very high level of clinical expertise and/or having responsibility for the planning of services.
9	More Senior Staff	Staff with the ultimate responsibility for clinical caseload decision-making and having full on-call accountability.

AGENDA FOR CHANGE

Agenda for Change is the most radical shake-up of the NHS pay system since the NHS began in 1948. It applies to over a million NHS staff with the exception of doctors, dentists and senior managers. Agenda for Change was implemented in the NHS across the UK on 1 December 2004 with pay, terms and conditions backdated to 1 October 2004. It involves a new NHS pay scheme which aims to provide a better means of rewarding staff for the application of additional knowledge and skills. Integral to Agenda for Change is the development of an NHS-wide Knowledge and Skills Framework (KSF) to underpin the new pay system, which emphasises the importance of personal development plans and recognises a shift to competency based learning.

The advantage of the new NHS pay scheme is that it offers appropriate levels of remuneration to nurses, midwives and professionals allied to medicine who undertake programmes of learning beyond registration in order to undertake specialist or advanced roles.

NATIONAL PRACTITIONER PROGRAMME

The National Practitioner Programme (NPP) in England encompasses a range of projects that focus on the delvelopment and mainstreaming of non-medical practitioner roles. The programme is continuing and furthering the work done by the Changing Workforce Programme which closed in March 2005 but which pioneered piloting role redesign to improve patient services.

The Changing Workforce Programme (CWP) as part of the NHS Modernisation Agency (England) was established in 2001 (Hargadon and Younger 2005). It was established to look at new ways of working to improve patient care, maximise the use of staff skills, tackle staff shortages and increase job satisfaction. The CWP has been responsible for supporting health and social care to redesign healthcare roles. In England various pilots were established to help determine how role redesign can improve service delivery and patient outcomes. Over 150 roles were developed and assessed for their impact on patient care, meeting the criteria that every role redesign is 'better for patients and better for staff'. The nursing and midwifery professions have been at the forefront of modernisation, taking on such responsibilities as nurse prescribing. The CWP has been instrumental in supporting projects that have addressed problems with the reduction in junior doctors' hours as a result of the European Working Time Regulations (EWTR) 1998. These include extending nursing and other healthcare practitioner roles, developing medical assessment facilities, introducing medical support workers and facilitating alternative night cover arrangements.

The Hospital at Night project has proven to be particularly successful, advocating that the best way to achieve care for patients at night is to have one or more multidisciplinary teams working in the hospital, who between them have the full range of skills to meet patients' immediate needs. The project redefined how medical cover is provided in hospitals during the out of hours period. The model consists of a multidisciplinary night team, which has the competencies to cover a wide range of interventions but has the capacity to call in specialist expertise when necessary. This contrasts with the traditional model of junior doctors working in relative isolation, and in specialty-based silos.

The project also advocates:

- supervised multi-specialty handover in the evenings;
- other staff taking on some of the work traditionally done by junior doctors;
- moving a significant proportion of non-urgent work from the night to the evening or daytime;
- reducing the unnecessary duplication of work by better coordination and reducing multiple clerking and reviews.

The rise of advanced nursing practitioners coincides with the reduction in junior doctors' working hours as a result of the EWTR. New nursing posts of Clinical Site Practitioners (CSPs) have been developed at Great Ormond Street Hospital for Children NHS Trust to address the shortage of junior doctors, especially at night (2004). The CSPs carry out regular ward rounds, assess sick children and are able to alter prescribed treatment regimes.

The CWP has acknowledged that at local and national level many new roles have been developed as part of the modernisation agenda. The proliferation of new roles resulted in pressure to develop a career framework so that skills, competencies and educational qualifications are transferable across the NHS. The outcome was the introduction of The Career Framework described above.

REGULATION AND PATIENT SAFETY

When roles are designed which cross professional boundaries it often raises questions of regulated practice. For registered staff who extend their scope of practice the current regulatory bodies, the Nursing Midwifery Council and Health Professions Council, provide codes of conduct so such staff are aware of their accountability and responsibilities when taking on new roles. In the absence of a regulatory body each employing organisation would need to ensure that staff such as assistant theatre or plaster practitioners are clearly aware of their responsibilities and accountability. This can be achieved by local contracts, policies and codes of conduct.

Many nurses and midwives have already embraced the modernisation agenda and have achieved role redesign supported by national policy initiatives such as the Chief Nursing Officer's 10 key roles for nurses, set out below.

Chief nursing officer's 10 key roles for nurses, 2000

1. To order diagnostic investigations such as pathology test and X-rays.
2. To make and receive referrals direct, say, to a therapist or pain consultant.
3. To admit and discharge patients for specified conditions and within agreed protocols.
4. To manage patient caseloads, say for diabetes or rheumatology.
5. To run clinics, say for ophthalmology or dermatology.
6. To prescribe medicines and treatments.
7. To carry out a wide range of resuscitation procedures including defibrillation.
8. To perform minor surgery and outpatient procedures.
9. To triage patients using the latest IT.

10. To take the lead in the way local health services are organised and the way that they are run.

One area of healthcare that has been responsive to patient need and the reduction of junior doctors' hours is that of perioperative care. Martin (2002) described how an extended role was developed to enable a nurse practitioner to undertake minor surgery in a nurse led clinic at St Mary's NHS Trust. A one stop service is provided with a see and treat facility offering patients a local service for the removal of minor skin lesions, sebaceous cysts and papillomas which are removed under local anaesthesia by a nurse practitioner. Facilitation of this service not only reduces waiting lists but prevents patients having to endure an outpatient appointment followed by a booked admission to a day surgery facility. In accordance with the aspirations of the NHS Plan 2000 the nurse practitioner post has been developed to provide integrated care for patients.

The experienced surgical nurse practitioner had already received validated training to assist the operating surgeon within the operating theatre under the direct supervision of the surgeon but was also provided with intensive training to enable the surgical nurse practitioner to perform minor surgical procedures independently. The outcome of this development is that waiting lists and waiting times have been reduced for the patient, junior doctors have been freed up to undertake other tasks whilst the nurse has extended her role and has job satisfaction. A new career pathway is available for non-medical personnel working within the perioperative environment through the development of a national surgical care practitioner curriculum (2005). Nurses and Operating Department Practitioners (ODPs) training and working as surgical care practitioners provide essential cover for doctors in training whose working week has been limited under the working time directive. In some organisations nurse practitioners have been trained to carry out simple hernia repairs.

The Perioperative Specialist Practitioner (PSP) is a new role enabling non-medical healthcare professionals to develop the skills, knowledge and competence needed to work alongside the Pre-Registration House Officers (PRHOs) and Senior House Officers (SHOs) in a surgical ward setting, carrying out duties such as preoperative assessment, admitting, clerking, history taking, preparing patients for surgery, postoperative management, discharge and follow-up.

Role redesign to improve patient outcomes has been significant with endoscopy. In March 2003, the CWP commenced a pilot for new ways of working in endoscopy at Castle Hill Hospital in Hull. Castle Hill developed a training programme for three individuals from different backgrounds to gain the knowledge and skills required to competently perform lower gastrointestinal endoscopy (sigmoidoscopy). One of these trainees was a direct entrant who trained to become an endoscopy technician. These practitioners perform this procedure on low risk patients having their own clinic in parallel with the consultant and seeking advice when required. The pilot has involved the training of practitioners from a variety of backgrounds to perform flexible sigmoidoscopy competently. Increasing the number of endoscopy practitioners is crucial if flexible sigmoidoscopy becomes part of the national routine bowel screening programme. With the additional practitioners flexible sigmoidoscopy waiting times have been reduced from five months to zero. Patients can have this investigation immediately rather than having to wait as they did in the past before role redesign.

The Emergency Nurse Practitioner (ENP) has been established for a number of years within the UK (Head 1988; Dealey 2001) and is recognised as improving the patient's care pathway through the A & E department. Walsh (1995) defines an ENP as 'A nurse who is practising in an autonomous but accountable way, providing care to patients independent of direct medical supervision'. The Audit Commission 2001 reported that waiting times in A & E were getting longer and recommended extending the scope of nursing practice by the introduction of emergency nurse practitioners.

Nurses working in accident and emergency (A & E) and critical care areas should be undertaking more medical functions according to the Department of Health and Royal College of Nurses (RCN) 2003 report *Freedom to Practise, Dispelling the Myths.* This report highlighted those unnecessary obstacles in relation to role boundaries that have prevented nurses expanding their roles into doctors' territory and recommended that these obstacles need to be removed if modernisation of the NHS is to be successful. The report outlined that nurses with the right competencies should be able to clerk and treat cardiology patients, order CT scans and blood results, refer patients and discharge patients from medical and surgical wards. Wintle (2005) has described how the CWP has developed the Emergency Care Practitioner (ECP) role to support the first contact needs of patients. This includes responding to emergency/urgent situations and carrying out appropriate interventions as necessary. ECPs are now working in urgent care centres where they can respond to 999 calls and undertake home visits.

WHAT'S IN A TITLE?

In recent years there has been a proliferation of titles especially in nursing and midwifery. Caroll (2002) recognised that there is much disagreement between academics, professional bodies and local NHS Trusts about the nature and expertise of levels of practice, in particular specialist and advanced practice.

There is currently a major debate within healthcare as to when a nurse can be deemed a specialist or an advanced practitioner. There appears to be little consensus about exactly what levels of skill, knowledge and experience should be required to attain a specialist title. There is an alarming lack of consistency as to when the title can be used. Nurses who have completed doctorates or a master's qualification will often call themselves specialists but then so could a nurse working in an Accident and Emergency department after in-house training. Clearly there needs to be some standardisation of the use of such titles to prevent confusion not only within the healthcare profession but also for patients.

The Nursing and Midwifery Council (Welsh Institute for Health and Social Care, 2004) commissioned the Welsh Institute for Health and Social Care to review the situation and outline a way forward. The institute discovered over 20 different practitioner or specialist titles being used with there often being very little difference between the titles. The NMC is consulting on this issue and favours a separate part of the register for such practitioners, together with a master's programme. The NMC is required by law to protect the public but does not currently have any standards in education and practice for many of the nurses that use the new titles.

In New Zealand this situation has been addressed by certain titles being protected and disciplinary action being taken against nurses who use them without permission, while the USA has minimum standards backed by law that must be attained by nurse practitioners educated to master's level. The USA also has core competencies for all nurse practitioner graduates. By contrast if you are a nurse practitioner in A & E you may have only done a five day course. Within the UK there are a range of courses and educational programmes to facilitate and support specialist practice. The Northern Ireland Practice and Education Council (NIPEC) facilitate over 250 courses to support specialist practice in Northern Ireland. Most courses have been developed through close working between NHS services and local academic providers.

Confusion regarding nursing titles is not only limited to patients but also affects other professionals outside the immediate team. There are currently a wide range of titles in use among post-registration nurses, including nurse practitioner, nurse clinician, highly specialised nurse, consultant nurse, clinical nurse specialist, and advanced nurse practitioner, to name but a few (WIHSC 2004). Such titles assume either a specialist or an advanced level of practice but apart from the new consultant roles many role developments have occurred in an ad hoc way largely in the absence of national guidance. A new level of registration for nursing is proposed by the NMC. The advanced role of the nurse practitioner may be recognised, where a master's level qualification underpins autonomous practice, differential diagnosis and prescribing of treatment.

The expansion of nursing and non-medical roles continues to increase and such role expansion must be welcomed if this trend is beneficial to patient care. Certainly never before has there been such scope for healthcare professionals to develop their practice or opportunities to take on what were previously designated medical tasks. It is important that such new roles are established strategically to ensure that they are clinically effective and are supported by appropriate validated training. When formulating a new job description and job specification this should be done in collaboration with the employer. The local Human Resource department can provide the expertise to ensure that the post holder will comply with the employing organisation's vicarious liability.

The debate as to whether nurse specialists are specialists more aligned to nursing or practitioners more closely aligned with medical roles is set to continue. Nursing as a science has seen a natural evolution in which boundaries have always been changing in order to enhance the quality of patient care. The ultimate question has to be 'what is in a title?' Ultimately what matters to patients is that whoever delivers care it is administered by a competent person with the right skills at the most convenient time. Political drivers such as the European Working Time Regulations (EWTR) are putting increasing pressures on healthcare organisations which have led to the increase in pilots developing new practitioner roles where nurse practitioner led clinics have reduced waiting times and provided new career opportunities. Some argue that this is nothing more than a stopgap for the shortage of doctors. The NHS has traditionally been predominantly medically focused but now it can be argued that the plethora of new nursing roles has ensured that nurses as a profession and practitioners working in professions allied to medicine have all added value to the specialisation of care which can only be of major benefit to the patient.

REFERENCES

The Audit Commission (2001) *Accident and Emergency Review of National Findings.* Wetherby: Audit Commission.

Carroll M (2002) Advancing nursing practice *Nursing Standard* **16** (29), 33–35.

Champions of advanced nursing practice (2004) *Professional Nurse* **19** (19), 20.

Dealey C (2001) Emergency Nurse Practitioners: should the role be developed? *British Journal of Nursing* **10** (22), 1458–1468.

Department of Health (1998) European Working Time Regulations. http://www.dh.gov.uk/workingtime.

Department of Health (2000a) *NHS Plan – A Plan For Investment – A Plan for Reform.* London: DH.

Department of Health (2000b) *A Health Service for all the Talents.* London: DH.

Department of Health (2000c) *NHS Plan – Chief Nursing Officer's Ten Key Roles for Nurses.* Cm 4848-1, 83–84. London: DH.

Department of Health (2000d) *Improving Working Lives.* London: DH.

Department of Health (2002) *Liberating the Talents: Helping Primary Care Trusts and Nurses to Deliver the NHS Plan.* London: DH.

Department of Health (2003) *Making a Difference: a First Class Service.* London: DH.

Department of Health (2004a) *Agenda for Change.* London: DH.

Department of Health (2004b) *The NHS Improvement Plan: Putting People at the Heart of Public Services.* London: DH.

Department of Health and Royal College of Nursing (2003) *Freedom to Practise: Dispelling the Myths.* London DH.

Developing Better Services: Modernising Hospitals and Reforming Structures in Northern Ireland (2002).

Hargadon J, Younger J (2005) Exploring new ways of working. *The Clinical Services Journal.* May: 16–19.

Head S (1988) The new pioneers *Nursing Times.* **84** (26), 27–28.

Martin S (2002) Cutting edge nursing *Nursing Times.* **98** (33), 22–23.

National Practitioner Programme. http://www.wise.nhs.uk/sites/workforce/practitioners.

NHS Modernisation Agency (2003) *Changing Workforce Programme: Pilot Sites Progress Report.*

NHS Modernisation Agency (2004) *A Career Framework for the NHS: Discussion Document* (version 2).

NHS Modernisation Agency *Changing Workforce Programme.* www.modern.nhs.uk/cwp.

NHS Modernisation Agency *Working Time Directive Pilots Programme: Hospitals at Night.* http://www.modern.nhs.uk/scripts/default.asp?site_id=50&id=17048

Post registration development: a framework for planning, commissioning and delivering learning beyond registration for nurses and midwive.: The report of a task group chaired by the CNO August 2004.

Scottish Executive (2000) *Our National Health: a New Agenda in Scotland.*

Scottish Executive (2004) National Workforce Plan for NHS Scotland.

Skills for Health Career Framework for Health Methodology Testing Report (2006) www.skillsforhealth.org.uk/careerframework.

Walsh M (1995) Nurse practitioners: Why are they so successful? *Emergency Nurse* **3** (2), 4–5.

Welsh Assembly (2001) *Improving Health: the NHS Plan for Wales.*

Welsh Institute for Health and Social Care (2004) *Innovation and Protection: A Framework for Post Registration.* Nursing report for the Nursing and Midwifery Council task force and Finish Group. School of Care Sciences, University of Glamorgan, Pontypridd.

Wintle C (2005) Redefining Emergency Care Roles *Clinical Services Journal* 58–60.

3 Training and Education

BARRY PARASKEVA

APPRECIATION OF SCOPE OF PRACTICE

Undertaking healthcare as a profession is married with an inherent responsibility for the safety and treatment of patients. In arenas where there is a significant interventional component, such as surgery, practitioners must approach their practice in a disciplined and systematic manner. Once the decision has been made to train within a surgical specialty you must appreciate the scope of your practice, understanding that you have the potential to cause harm as well as good to patients. The risks associated with surgery can be overcome with robust training systems with regular mentoring and assessment of practice. When undertaking training candidates must undertake thorough training which will be both rewarding and disappointing along the way, and accept constructive criticism from tutors as well as carrying out a great deal of self-analysis. After a decision has been made to train as a minor surgical practitioner there are certain steps you need to consider in your training before you embark. These are:

- selection of institution;
- adequate mentoring;
- educational modalities;
- methods of assessment;
- record keeping and audit;
- applying theory to independent practice.

SELECTION OF INSTITUTION

The selection of the institution for training is critical in furthering your experience, as a wrong decision at this stage can lead to disillusionment and ultimately failure to reach goals. Many independent surgical practitioners have a previous medical background, usually nursing. It follows that the majority

Minor Surgical Procedures for Nurses and Allied Healthcare Professionals. Edited by Shirley Martin.
© 2007 John Wiley & Sons Limited

of nurses who become surgical practitioners are those that have been exposed to surgery before in their clinical job, either as scrub nurses, working in endoscopy, surgical wards or accident and emergency. It also is common for many well established clinical staff to take on new roles within their base hospitals, usually due to new initiatives within departments leading to improved opportunities. With increasing interest by government and the NHS in developing new practitioner roles there is a demand for standardisation of training, proformas of practice, and the provision of centres with established courses and facilities to educate larger numbers of students. Therefore, when selecting an institution the student must consider which have the best opportunities for training, established teaching courses and facilities, and a proven track record in the area.

Institutions that offer structured training and clinical exposure are essential to successful development. There needs to be a free and easy dialogue between students and their teachers, usually surgical clinicians. The institution should ideally have a clinical skills laboratory, where seminars and skills sessions can be run at regular intervals, and which can also be the setting for examination and assessment.

Clinical experience is of vital importance once you have undergone the initial training, hence your chosen institution must provide exposure to patients, operating potential, ability to attend clinics and 'see and treat' sessions. Inadequate clinical opportunities will lead to a deterioration in confidence and boredom, since the overall goal is putting theory into practice. To achieve this goal the academic functions of an institution must be in harmony with the policies of the Trust involved, which needs to be interested and willing to fund and support practitioner training schemes.

Adequate mentoring

Learning practical skills requires supervision. Although a great deal can be learnt from books, videos, the internet and interactive programmes, craft specialties are best taught by a mentor. It is envisaged that as the interest in training surgical practitioners increases, the number of dedicated tutors will expand to meet this demand. If you are in an institution where your clinical work is based, it is easier to approach people you trust and whom you know have an interest in education. The relationship is crucial to development. If clinicians are used as mentors, regular meeting times need to be arranged, although there has to be a degree of flexibility also. Your mentor should not only teach you but also regularly assess you and give you constructive criticism with sets of goals for you to aim at prior to the next session. It is also preferable if your chosen mentor is a surgeon, who could then take you to relevant theatre lists and directly supervise your involvement in clinical cases. The surgeon can also provide advice on difficult cases and management decisions; and can also be called upon if complications occur during surgical procedures.

EDUCATIONAL MODALITIES

As mentioned earlier, it is important to have a trusted surgical mentor in an institution which is interested in training surgical practitioners and has the facilities and funding to do so.

In general performing surgical procedures requires the following.

- Adequate anatomical knowledge of the tissues and structures likely to be encountered.
- Knowledge of relevant physiology and pharmacology of agents that you are likely to use in practice, eg local anaesthetic agents.
- Clinical skills practice, which should be a repetitive process with a mentor, preceded by learning and preparation from books/manuals, videos or inter-active/web-based programmes.
- Clinical exposure. Initially this should be with a mentor, and should take the form of sitting in clinics and minor operating sessions and assisting in the main operating theatre, as this will allow you to put learnt skills into practice, such as suturing. This will improve your knowledge of tissue hand-ling. Another vital component of clinical exposure is the assessment of the student's communication skills. This skill is very important as the practi-tioner has to inspire confidence in the patient, obtain the necessary clinical information prior to surgery, and explain the procedure with clarity so that informed consent may be given.
- It is of vital importance to keep an accurate log of all the procedures you have learnt, how many procedures you have seen, how many of them you have assisted at and how many you have performed.

Within a dedicated training unit it would be envisaged that all of the above would be available to students.

There are many widely available sources for the study of operative practice. There are books and manuals that describe the principles involved in operat-ing. Video/DVD and internet-based teaching material allows a more ani-mated and on occasion interactive educational experience. The majority of initial technique work is undertaken within the setting of skills laboratories with the use of bench top models such as rubber suture pads. Try to use the same instruments in the lab situation as you would use clinically, and always approach procedural practice as you would a real case, taking care with instruments and tissue handling, always keeping sterility in mind.

In addition to your institutional training there are now increasing numbers of courses in basic surgical skills and operative theatre assisting which are certificated and assist in evaluation and accreditation.

METHODS OF ASSESSMENT

After periods of training students need to be assessed to see whether they are competent or not. What defines competent depends on the criteria laid down. However, in the main the most important factors are the ability to advise the correct management, execute the procedure safely and understand your own limitations, knowing when assistance is required.

There are many ways to assess practitioners. None of the currently available methods is exclusive, and different types of assessment are used for differing aspects of practice. The basic knowledge aspects of practice, for example anatomy, pathology and pharmacology, can easily be assessed using a multiple choice paper or, now becoming increasingly popular, the extended matching question paper, in which students must match the most appropriate answers to clinical scenarios. It is also of value for students to prepare longer term research-based dissertations, for which they need to study and investigate an aspect of surgical practice as a project.

Assessment of surgical skill is of increasing importance across the clinical arena to ensure a level of baseline competency. There have been problems in introducing assessment tools as there needs to be an objective non-biased way of performing these assessments. For the assessment of practitioner skill, there should be regular reviews by mentors to guide development and spot potential problems early. However, for the purposes of accreditation a more formal assessment is usually required. Of increasing popularity is the Objective Structured Clinical Examination (OSCE) format, where all students undertake the same sets of standardised tasks. which are objectively scored by examiners.

As mentioned previously, communication is of vital importance. This can be assessed by placing students in a clinical scenario with simulated patients with the consultation being videoed, allowing not only assessment but analysis and advice from mentors. It is now possible to combine mock skills stations (OSCEs) with a communication aspect which gives a more realistic scenario.

The other aspects of assessment concern continued evaluation while in clinical practice and review of cases performed to form a portfolio.

RECORD KEEPING

It is essential for educational and medico-legal purposes that you keep a comprehensive record of the cases you have performed in a logbook. It is also advisable to use digital pictures of before and after surgery and also pictures of any complications of your practice. Some practitioners even video their cases. A suggested approach is to create a case folder for each of the patients you see and operate on. This will contain evidence of your evaluation of the patient and also the consent form which the patient has to sign in a fully informed manner. It will also show that the procedure has been explained, and provide evidence that the patient understands you are a practitioner and is happy to be treated by you.

In your case notes you should have proformas which could be in the form of a booklet on which can be recorded clinical and operative details. After the patient is discharged you should follow them up in the community with a phone call and chase relevant histology results, as some of your patients will need further evaluation and treatment. Keeping a log in this fashion allows the results to be presented for review to mentors, assessors and members of the hospital Trusts to allow accreditation and the granting of a contract for independent practice. The accurate keeping of records, assisted by the use of electronic databases, allows audit of your practice by yourself and others which can lead to improvements and changes in working practices.

Applying theory to independent practice

The goal is to have adequate knowledge and competency to practise independently. However, it must be appreciated that even when accredited the majority of practitioners are still learning. As such there will be times of difficulty, made increasingly stressful when you are an independent practitioner. Your clinical practice needs to be carried out within the context of a structured well documented framework, with adequate audit and support, both academically from mentors and from hospital Trusts. Increasing confidence will come with time, allowing you to embark on more challenging clinical cases.

The development of a competent and safe surgical practitioner is a long process reliant on a defined structure of training, support from medical and academic staff, and excellent documentation for audit purposes. The future has arrived and the concept of surgical practitioners is no longer new. To increase numbers and improve training the way forward is to develop accredited teaching courses that can cope with all the needs of larger cohorts of surgical practitioners.

4 Nurse Prescribing

ANN CLARRIDGE

One of the most significant recent developments within the National Health Service (NHS) in the United Kingdom has been the emergence of prescribing by healthcare professionals other than doctors or dentists. The NHS Plan (Department of Health 2000b) and Liberating the Talents (Department of Health 2002a) are concerned with the development of nurses' roles and the use of their skills to improve the health of the population, with the nurse prescriber as one of the 10 key roles within the NHS Plan.

This chapter seeks to address a number of different issues in relation to nurse prescribing. It will address:

- the background and history of nurse prescribing;
- the different categories of nurse prescribing and the options available to nurses in order for them to complete an episode of care experienced by a patient including Patient Group Directions (PGDs);
- the implications of nurse prescribing in practice;
- the legal framework and accountability of nurse prescribing;
- the education and preparation for nurse prescribing.

BACKGROUND TO THE DEVELOPMENT OF NURSE PRESCRIBING

In the Neighbourhood Nursing Review (Cumberlege Report, DHSS 1986) it was suggested that experienced district nurses working in the community were wasting their valuable time waiting outside general practitioners' doorways for prescriptions for clients whom they had already assessed and diagnosed without the involvement of the medical practitioner. The report recommended that qualified community nurses should be able to prescribe from a limited formulary. An advisory group under the leadership of Dr June Crown was set up to review the necessary arrangements for nurses to be able to prescribe. The recommendations from the review (DHSS 1986) proposed that a limited list of items could be prescribed by nurses with a District Nurse (DN) or Health Visitor (HV) qualification with an additional recognition that in the future it

Minor Surgical Procedures for Nurses and Allied Healthcare Professionals. Edited by Shirley Martin.
© 2007 John Wiley & Sons Limited

might be possible to extend the formulary and prescribing rights to other groups of nurses. The United Kingdom Central Council (UKCC) and the English National Board for Nurses, Midwives and Health Visitors (ENB) developed a limited formulary of medicines, appliances and dressings. The *Nurse Prescribers' Formulary (NPF)* comprised those items highlighted as being most useful for district nurses and health visitors and included such items as are used in the management of wounds, constipation, scabies and threadworms, head louse infections, urinary incontinence and mild to moderate pain.

The practice context for nurse prescribing

The Government's policy in expanding nurse prescribing powers aims to enable patients to access medicines quickly and safely while making optimal use of professional knowledge and skills.

Consider a number of healthcare settings in which nurses may find themselves working:

- walk-in centre;
- nurse led clinic for sexually transmitted diseases;
- general practice nurse running a minor injuries and minor illness clinic;
- nurse practitioner running a chronic disease clinic for patients with, for example, asthma or diabetes;
- nurse in secondary care running a clinic for patients with, for example, Parkinson's disease, diabetes, skin disorders;
- community mental health outreach clinic.

In each of these different areas of professional practice nurses may be working independently of a medical practitioner and where a doctor is not immediately available. The options available to the nurse will depend on the kind of education and training they have undertaken for prescribing. They may prescribe as:

- an Independent Prescriber from the *Community Practitioners' Formulary* (NMC 2006). This was formerly known as the *Nurse Prescribers' Formulary for District Nurses and Health Visitors*;
- an Independent Extended Nurse Prescriber from the *Extended Nurse Prescribers' Formulary (ENPF)*; and/or
- as a Supplementary Prescriber within the framework of a Clinical Management Plan.

Independent prescribers are defined as 'professionals who are responsible for the initial assessment of the patient and for devising the broad treatment plan, with the authority to prescribe the medicines required as part of that plan' (Department of Health 1999).

Supplementary prescribing is defined as 'a voluntary partnership between an independent prescriber (a doctor or dentist) and a supplementary prescriber to implement an agreed patient-specific Clinical Management Plan (CMP) with the patient's agreement' (Department of Health 2003b).

NURSE PRESCRIBING AND PATIENT GROUP DIRECTIONS CLARIFIED

There is a need to emphasise the difference between the terms 'prescribing' and 'supply and administration' of medicines. The prescriber makes a choice regarding the medication to be taken by the patient in concordance with them and based on their initial assessment of the patient. The prescriber then issues a prescription which is a legal order requesting the supply of a medicine and which also gives instructions how the medicine should be administered. The medication has to be supplied or administered exactly as advised on the prescription.

In a healthcare setting where the patient may not be individually identified before presenting for treatment a medicine can be supplied or administered under a PGD, for example in immunisations or emergency contraception. A PGD is drawn up locally by doctors, pharmacists and other health professionals and must meet certain legal criteria (DH 2005). Nurses are able to supply and administer Prescription Only Medicines (POMs) in accordance with Patient Group Directions (PGDs) formerly known as Group Protocols but this is not prescribing.

PATIENT GROUP DIRECTIONS (PGDS)

In the early stages of the development of PGDs previously known as Group Protocols the law regarding their use was somewhat grey; however, there are a number of Statutory Instruments in place now that form the legislative framework for the use of PGDs in Great Britain. The instructions for the use of PGDs are given in the HSC 2000/026 (England), WHC (2000)116 (Wales), and HDL2001(7) (Scotland). PGDs deal with the situation, not the individual patient. It is important to distinguish between prescribing for an individual patient and supplying and administering a medicine for a group of patients under an agreed PGD. A PGD may be restrictive in the choice of medication that can be supplied or administered by the non-medical professional using them, however, they are written for a medicine or a group of medicines in very exacting terms and therefore no other medicine dose or regimes can be used. Typically nurses currently use PGDs for the supply and administration of flu vaccination, travel vaccination and emergency contraception, although this list is by no means exhaustive.

LEGAL FRAMEWORK

The necessary legislation that enables nurse prescribing was provided in the Medicines Products: Prescribing by nurses, etc., Act, 1992. The Act came into force in 1994 enabling DNs and HVs to prescribe from the *Nurse Prescribers' Formulary*. The Government later expanded the range of conditions that nurses were able to prescribe for and broadened the range of products to meet the therapeutic requirements for those conditions. This extended formulary was referred to as the *Nurse Prescribers' Extended Formulary (NPEF)*. A list of all the conditions and preparations available may be found in the *British National Formulary (BNF)*. Supplementary prescribing allows those practitioners who can demonstrate the competencies required to prescribe from the whole of the *BNF* as identified within the Clinical Management Plan (CMP). Initially there were exceptions that related to the prescribing of controlled drugs and unlicensed drugs, unless the unlicensed drugs are used in clinical trials (Department of Health 2003b).

Section 63 of the Health and Social Care Act 2001 enabled the Government to extend prescribing responsibilities to other health professions and included the concept of supplementary prescriber. The Prescription Only Medicines Order and NHS regulations, allowing suitably trained nurses to become supplementary prescribers, was amended in 2003 (Department of Health 2003b).

On 14 April 2005 amendments to the Misuse of Drugs Regulations 2001 to enable nurse and pharmacist supplementary prescribers to prescribe controlled drugs and unlicensed medicines came into effect (DH 2005).

The supplementary prescriber is able to respond to the patients' therapeutic requirements without necessarily referring them back to the independent prescriber at each visit providing that the supplementary prescriber is working within the agreed CMP. In this way the supplementary prescriber is not limited to a particular condition or to a particular formulary, but rather is able to prescribe from the whole of the *BNF*. In secondary care supplementary prescribing appears to be linked normally to the nurse's clinical specialty (Erskine and Nuttan 2003; Bellingham 2004; Green 2004; James 2004). Supplementary prescribing has enormous potential for those nurses working in nurse-led clinics without ready access to a doctor.

The NMC has suggested that although nurses and midwives are now able to prescribe any medicine for any medical condition within their scope of practice and competence (DH 2006), supplementary prescribing may still be used under certain circumstances especially if they wish to prescribe from a full range of controlled drugs (NMC 2006).

ACCOUNTABILITY IN PRESCRIBING

Accountability in prescribing as in other areas of nursing practice means that the nurse prescriber is answerable to the patient and also to the employing organisations, colleagues, the NMC and the law. Nurse prescribing is a new skill and once qualified the nurse prescriber will be authorised to make a prescribing decision and will therefore be both legally and professionally accountable for all aspects of the decision-making process. This process includes the initial consultation, choice to prescribe or not, choice of treatment, advice given to the patient or carer, including information regarding the administration of medication, and subsequent treatment reviews.

Legally, there are several statutory documents that define the framework of law for nurse prescribing. The Medicinal Products: Prescribing by Nurses, etc., Act 1992 enabled nurses to prescribe from the limited *NPF*. The prescribing rights were expanded by the Health and Social Care Act 2001 and the amendments to the Medicines Orders and NHS Regulations that enabled prescribing from the *NPEF* and, subsequently, the implementation of supplementary prescribing and later to prescribe any medicine for any medical condition within their scope of practice and level of competence (DH 2006; NMC 2006). Any form of breach of the enactments of the Medicines Act 1968 and other relevant legislation makes the prescriber liable to prosecution. It is crucial therefore that the nurse prescriber is familiar with NMC guidance on 'standards of conduct that nurses, midwives and specialist community public health nurses are required to meet in their level of expertise and their practice as a registered prescriber' and recognises the challenge this presents to ensure that they prescribe within their area of competence.

EDUCATION

Historically the ENB developed a short course curriculum, Mode 1, V100, for the education and training of district nurses and health visitors in 1992. Successful completion of the two day taught course comprising basic pharmacology, accountability and prescribing safely and effectively, would qualify them as nurse prescribers. It is now the practice (Mode 2, V200) to incorporate the learning outcomes for the prescribing programme for District Nurses and Health Visitors into the Specialist Practitioner Programme. DNs and HVs now only qualify as a Specialist Practitioner upon successful completion of the prescribing component of the programme. As mentioned earlier, the ENB and the subsequent Nursing and Midwifery Council for England (NMC) devised a number of learning outcomes and a curriculum to meet the education and training needs for District Nurses and Health Visitors to prescribe from the limited formulary. In order to prepare nurses to prescribe from the *Nurse Prescribers' Extended Formulary* a programme was devised comprising 25 days of contact time for the theory component, plus 12 days of practice during which a designated medical practitioner supervises the practitioner. This programme was extended by two days to accommodate the additional learning outcomes required for supplementary prescribing. Higher Education institutions are offering a combined programme so that nurses who have successfully undertaken the programme can have the qualification of V300 recorded against their name with the NMC as recognition that they are qualified to prescribe from the *ENPF* and as a supplementary prescriber.

THE CHALLENGES FACING NURSES IN RELATION TO PRESCRIBING

It is important to identify the 'right' mode of prescribing for your area of practice and for you. Think about your area of practice and the options available and what this means in terms of your further education and training needs. The level of knowledge of pharmacology and pharmacotherapeutics required in order to prescribe competently and safely is significantly more than is currently taught in pre-registration programmes.

The skill of critical appraisal is crucial to ensuring effective and safe practice and is a requirement within the Government's Clinical Governance agenda.

Medicines are constantly changing; therefore it is important to maintain practice in line with new developments and current research. It is vital to maintain competence as a practitioner through regular updating and the use of evidence-based guidelines produced by the National Institute for Health and Clinical Excellence and the National Service Frameworks for the relevant area of practice.

A large proportion of medication is not taken or used by patients; achieving concordance is time consuming but cost effective in the long term. There is a need to recognise the 'expert patient'.

Team working can be difficult with different levels of skills and expertise, and can be confusing for patients, who may be presented with various opinions from different professionals. Therefore there is a need to collaborate and share good practice to ensure effective, safe patient care.

DEVELOPMENTS IN PRESCRIBING

One of the recommendations in the Crown Report 11 (Department of Health 1999b) was to extend supplementary prescribing to new groups of healthcare professionals in order to better utilise the skills and abilities of the NHS workforce. Since April 2003, pharmacists have been able to undertake further education and training to become supplementary prescribers and on 14 April 2005 changes to the regulations came into effect to enable radiographers and other allied health professionals to become supplementary prescribers. On 1 May 2006 further changes came into force enabling nurse independent prescribing and pharmacist independent prescribing as detailed earlier in this chapter. Higher Education institutions will offer flexible programmes to prepare all these practitioners from different professional disciplines, together with nurses. The programmes will be designed to meet the different professional needs as well as offering opportunities for shared learning.

CONCLUSION

Crucial to prescribing, supply and administration of medicines through PGDs is the need for adequate and appropriate education to achieve safe, competent practice. At the same time it is of paramount importance that practitioners maintain their competence throughout their professional careers. The delivery of high quality healthcare based on the best available evidence is a key aspect of the Government's modernisation agenda (Department of Health 2002b). Most obviously, prescribing by nurses is an exciting but challenging development in their professional history but it is not without risks and the nurse needs to be aware of this.

A successful student and now a practising nurse prescriber remarked, 'I am now more aware of all aspects of the information required before I make any prescribing decisions, but it is so worth while when I know that I can complete the care for the patient'. This statement encapsulates the benefits of the new prescribing agenda for nurses.

REFERENCES AND FURTHER READING

Bellingham C (2004) How supplementary prescribing helps in both acute and chronic hospital care. *Pharmaceutical Journal* **272** (22), 640–641.

British Medical Association & Royal Pharmaceutical Society of Great Britain (2004) *British National Formulary*. Oxford: Pharmaceutical Press.

Clarridge A, Ryder E (2004) Working collaboratively. In (eds Chilton S, Melling K, Drew D, Clarridge A) *Nursing in the Community An Essential Guide to Practice*. London: Arnold.

Department of Health (DH) (1968) *HMG Medicines Act*. London: Stationery Office.

Department of Health (1989) *Report of the Advisory Group on Nurse Prescribing*. London: DH.

Department of Health (1992) *The Medicines Products: Prescribing by Nurses, etc., Act*. London: Stationery Office.

Department of Health (1997), *A Report on the Supply and Administration of Medicines Under Group Protocols* (Crown Report I). London: Stationery Office.

Department of Health (1999a) *Saving Lives: Our Healthier* Nation. London: Stationery Office.

Department of Health (1999b) *Review of Prescribing, Administration and Supply of Medicines*. Final Report (Crown Report II). London: Stationery Office.

Department of Health (2000a) Health Service Circular 2000/026. London: DH.

Department of Health (2000b) *The NHS Plan: a Plan for Investment, a Plan for Reform*. London: DH.

Department of Health (2001) *The Health and Social Care Act*. London: DH.

Department of Health (2002a) *Liberating the Talents. Helping Primary Care Trusts and Nurses to Deliver the NHS Plan*. London: DH.

Department of Health (2002b) *Extending Independent Nurse Prescribing Within the NHS in England: a Guide for Implementation*. London: DH.

Department of Health (2003a) *A Vision for Pharmacy in the New NHS*, London: DH.

Department of Health (2003b) *Supplementary Prescribing by Nurses and Pharmacists Within the NHS in England. A guide for implementation.* London: DH.

Department of Health (2004a) *Extending Independent Nurse Prescribing Within the NHS in England. A Guide for Implementation* (2nd edn). London: DH.

Department of Health (2004b) *HSC 1999/065. Clinical Governance in the New NHS.* London: DH.

Department of Health (2004c) More health professionals to be given power to prescribe. Press Release 2004/0179, Media Centre. London: DH.

Department of Health (2005) Summary of changes to regulations on supplementary prescribing. Ref number: Gateway reference 4912.

Department of Health (2006) *Medicines Matter: A Guide to Mechanisms for the Prescribing, Supply and Administration of Medicines.* London: DH.

Department of Health and Social Security (1986) *Neighbourhood Nursing: a Focus for Care* (Cumberlege Report). London: Stationery Office.

English National Board for Nurses, Midwives and Health Visitors (1992) *Nurse Prescribing: Background Briefing.* London: English National Board for Nurses, Midwives and Health Visitors.

Erskine D, Nuttan T (2003) *Supplementary Prescribing: Models Developing Within the UK Primary Care Setting.*

Green H (2004) Nurse prescribing in the acute sector: one Trust's experience. *Nurse Prescribing* **2** (1), 9–14.

Home Office Circular (2003) HOC 049/2003 Controlled drugs legislation – Nurse prescribing and patient group directions.

James J (2004) Supplementary prescribing by a diabetes specialist nurse on a hospital ward. *Nurse Prescribing* **2** (3), 112–116.

National Prescribing Centre (2001) *Maintaining competency in prescribing. An outline framework to help nurse prescribers* (1st edn). Liverpool: National Prescribing Centre.

Nursing and Midwifery Council (2002a) The Council's requirements for 'Extended Independent Nurse prescribing' and 'Supplementary Prescribing'. NMC Circular 25/2002. London: Nursing and Midwifery Council.

Nursing and Midwifery Council (2002b) *The NMC Code of Professional Conduct: Standards for Conduct, Performance and Ethics.* London: Nursing and Midwifery Council.

Nursing and Midwifery Council (2006) *Standards of Proficiency for Nurse and Midwife Prescribers.* London: NMC.

Robinson P (2005) *Non-Medical Prescribing: Changes to Regulations* MPIG-CCE. London: DH.

Thyer A, Robinson P (2004) *Proposals for Supplementary Prescribing by Chiropodists, Physiotheraists, Radiographers, and Optometrists and Proposed Amendments to the Prescription Only Medicines (Human Use) Order, 1997.* London: DH.

United Kingdom Central Council (1991) The Council's response to the Department of Health invitation to establish the standard, kind and content of educational preparation for nurse prescribing. MW/GM/8.107. London: United Kingdom Central Council.

United Kingdom Central Council (2001) Registrar's letter 28/2001. The Council's requirements for the standard, kind and content of educational programme for registered nurses, midwifes and health visitors to prescribe from the extended nurses prescriber's formulary. London: United Kingdom Central Council.

Weiss M, Britten N (2003) What is concordance? *British Medical Journal.* **327,** 856–858.

5 Medico-Legal Aspects of Non-Medical Practitioner Roles

VERITY DANZIGER

INTRODUCTION

Enhanced roles in nursing have changed the face of service delivery within the NHS. This chapter considers the legal issues surrounding the provision of care and treatment both generally and specifically in relation to enhanced roles. It is by no means an exhaustive guide to the law and is intended as an introduction only to selected parts of the legal framework of clinical practice and, in particular, the following.

1. Civil liability – the law relating to clinical negligence.
2. Consent.
3. NMC Guidelines.

1. CIVIL LIABILITY – THE LAW OF CRIMINAL NEGLIGENCE

1.1 CRIMINAL AND CIVIL LIABILITY

Criminal and civil liabilities are often confused. Criminal law is the way in which the state controls individual behaviour. The state sets rules that society must follow. If those rules are broken, a crime is committed and the state brings criminal proceedings on society's behalf in the criminal courts. If convicted, the state punishes the perpetrator of the crime.

Criminal proceedings against healthcare practitioners are not that common but practitioners could be involved in cases relating to the assault or manslaughter or murder. In the clinical context, healthcare is not an assault as long as the patient has consented to the treatment, and the crucial concept of

Minor Surgical Procedures for Nurses and Allied Healthcare Professionals. Edited by Shirley Martin.
© 2007 John Wiley & Sons Limited

consent is considered in section 2. It is important to note that the same act (for example surgery without a patient's consent), could lead to a civil claim for compensation as well as criminal prosecution for assault.

Civil law governs relationships between individuals and provides a remedy for an individual whose rights have been affected by the conduct of another. A patient who suffers an injury because of poor quality healthcare will bring a claim in the civil courts for financial compensation for clinical negligence.

1.2 INDEMNITY: WHOM DO PATIENTS SUE?

The NHS indemnity makes NHS bodies themselves rather than the individual practitioner legally liable for any negligent acts and omissions of their employees. NHS indemnity applies where the NHS body owed a duty of care to the patient and usually arises where: the negligent healthcare professional was working under a contract of employment (ie not a contract for services) and the negligence occurred in the course of that employment; or the negligent healthcare professional, although not working under a contract of employment, was contracted to an NHS body to provide services to persons to whom that NHS body owed a duty of care.

The NHS indemnity applies to all healthcare professionals including hospital doctors, dentists, nurses, midwives, health visitors and pharmacy practitioners, etc. The effect of the indemnity is that patients bring one set of proceedings against the NHS body rather than separate claims against, for example, one nurse in respect of alleged negligent prescribing and another nurse in respect of postoperative monitoring. The NHS Trust will be the sole defendant.

There are significant exceptions to what is covered by NHS indemnity and these include:

- a healthcare professional's private practice;
- disciplinary proceedings by statutory bodies such as the NMC;
- 'Good Samaritan' acts (eg assisting at the roadside at a traffic accident) and all actions taken outside the healthcare professional's work for the NHS employing body;
- independent midwives;
- criminal proceedings.

Some agency work may not be covered by the indemnity.

It is always advisable to clarify the professional indemnity position and to ensure that appropriate cover is in place for all professional activities in the event of a claim. The NMC specifically recommends that nurses have professional indemnity cover and that, if they do not, then this fact and its implications should be made clear to patients/clients.

1.3 THE LAW OF CLINICAL NEGLIGENCE

The general position is that, to establish liability in negligence, there must be a duty of care which is breached and which results in loss or damage to the patient. Considering each of these three ingredients in turn:

1.3.1 Is there a duty of care owed to the person treated by the relevant professional?

The existence of a duty of care is not usually a barrier to clinical negligence claims as it is inherent in the relationship between clinicians and patients.

1.3.2 Was there a breach of the duty of care by the professional not attaining the appropriate standard of care?

Clinical negligence is the provision of care or treatment that does not comply with reasonably competent clinical practice. This standard – of reasonable competence – has remained largely unchanged since a 1957 case *[Bolam* v *Friern Hospital Management Committee]* about a man who was injured in the course of ECT treatment and alleged that the safety measures were inadequate. The judge said:

> 'The test is the standard of the ordinary skilled man exercising and expressing to have that special skill. A doctor is not guilty of negligence if he has acted in accordance with a practice accepted as proper by a responsible body of medical men skilled in that particular art.'

To determine whether treatment complied with the expected standard, judges in clinical negligence cases will hear evidence from independent practitioners. General surgeons will advise on treatment provided by general surgeons and treatment provided by those in enhanced nursing roles should be commented on by professionals in the same field. While appropriately experienced medico-legal experts are still rather thin on the ground, that should change as the nursing role continues to expand. These independent experts advise the court about the treatment that can be expected from practitioners in the field – not about the expert's own practice and not about best practice but about the treatment that would represent reasonable practice.

A claim that involves enhanced nursing roles might involve the following allegations.

- It was inappropriate for the particular treatment to be provided by a nurse.
- The nurse departed from guidance or protocols in the provision of treatment.
- The nurse failed to seek medical guidance in a situation where it was required.
- The treatment provided did not in some other way comply with reasonably competent nurse practice.

Whether or not the patient has a successful claim will always depend on the facts. If there is national or local guidance covering a particular step, then this should usually be followed. If the guidance itself is thought to be either flawed or inappropriate for the particular circumstances, this should be brought to the attention of senior clinicians and the ensuing discussion about the treatment of an individual patient should be carefully noted. Guidelines (as opposed to protocols) are often not intended to be mandatory and are not intended to replace clinical judgment. All the same, departures from guidance will need to be carefully considered (and documented) if they are to be justified.

Many areas of enhanced practice are governed by strict protocols which are intended to be mandatory. Nurses in enhanced roles must ensure that they are familiar with any statutory framework that applies, such as that relating to requesting X-rays or prescribing, as well as any national and local protocols. Departures from a protocol, for example, providing treatment that is not covered by it or providing treatment to a patient who does not fit the protocol criteria, will be difficult to defend and, again, if there is concern about the application of a protocol to a particular patient, senior clinicians should be involved and the discussion should be noted in the records. Such departures increase the risk of clinical negligence proceedings as well as disciplinary proceedings.

Ultimately, the court will hear experts for the patient and for the NHS body. The judge has the ultimate power to scrutinise the evidence and decide whether the care provided stands up to logical analysis even if that care reflects relatively common practice.

1.3.3 Did the patient suffer loss or damage as a result of the breach of duty?

A patient can only recover damages if their injuries occurred as a result of the breach of duty. The crucial question is whether the injury would have happened 'but for' the negligence.

If the injury would have occurred anyway because, for example, of the patient's underlying condition, there is no claim. In one case, a hospital A & E department failed to diagnose arsenic poisoning and sent a patient home and he died later. However, the court accepted that the patient would have died even if his condition had been promptly diagnosed and treated. The claim failed because the patient's death was caused by the poison not the negligence.

Patients must establish that, on the balance of probabilities (ie a greater than 50% chance), their injury would have been avoided 'but for' the negligence. In a case where a child fell from a tree and sustained a fracture and then avascular necrosis, he had to establish that the avascular necrosis resulted from the hospital's delay in diagnosing the fracture rather than the fracture itself. However, the evidence was that there was a 75% chance that the avascular necrosis would have developed anyway so that claim failed because the patient did not show that the negligence had probably caused the damage.

1.4 THE ANATOMY OF A LEGAL CLAIM

1.4.1 Timescales

The basic rule is that patients have three years from the date of injury to bring a claim but there are exceptions including:

- where the patient is a child, the three years begin on the child's 18th birthday;
- where the patient is incapable of managing their own affairs;
- where there was a delay before the patient realised or could reasonably have found out that they had suffered an injury related to their treatment.

Once there is a claim, it passes through a pre-action phase as well as formal legal proceedings on its way to a trial. The pre-action phase involves the following steps.

- The patient obtains a copy set of their records and investigates (with the help of independent medical experts) the merits of the claim.
- The patient prepares a Letter of Claim setting out the facts of the case and the allegations to be pursued.
- The defendant then has three months to investigate the allegations and to provide a formal Letter of Response, making clear which allegations are conceded and which remain in dispute.

The claim may reach a conclusion in the pre-action stage either if the claimant is satisfied with the defendant's response or because the defendant admits liability and the parties are able to negotiate an appropriate settlement. Otherwise, the steps in formal proceedings include:

- the Claimant serves a Claim Form and Particulars of Claim, formally setting out the case to answer;
- the NHS body serves a Defence setting out its formal position;
- the parties exchange lists of all the documents relevant to the issues in the case;
- the parties exchange factual statements from the people (patients and clinicians) who were involved in the incident in question;
- the parties exchange reports from the relevant experts who have been instructed. The experts for both sides will also meet to see what issues can be agreed and what remains in dispute;

- the parties set out their positions in relation to the value of the claim in a Schedule of Loss and a Counter Schedule.

Once the evidence has been exchanged, there will be a trial and all the factual and expert witnesses will come to court and the judge will decide the result. Even when they are up and running, clinical claims can still take a long time to reach resolution. This can be because some medico-legal experts have waiting lists of many months for reports, and delays also arise when the prognosis of injured patients is unclear as this makes it difficult to arrive at an accurate valuation of the claim. This can take years where the claim is on behalf of a young child with a brain injury.

1.4.2 How are damages calculated?

Patients are entitled to compensation for problems that result from the below standard care, but not for problems that they would have sustained in any event. For example, if a fracture repair has been done badly, the claimant will be compensated for the consequences of the poor treatment but not for the original fracture and its likely *sequelae.*

There are two elements to an award. The first – general damages – compensates the patient for 'pain, suffering and loss of amenity'. The award varies from about £4000 for an unnecessary laparotomy scar to about £200000 for quadriplegia.

The remainder of any award is wholly related to the financial losses and extra expenses caused by the injury. So, if patients are unable to work or need care or equipment or physiotherapy, those direct financial losses form part of their claim.

1.4.3 Role of the clinician

It is worth emphasising the role of good notes in defending claims. There are very many cases where the quality of the notes either casts doubt on the quality of care or where the care provided and the reasons for it are unclear. For example, there may have been a departure from a particular treatment guideline but, if the records do not explain what was done and why, the departure may prove difficult to defend. The best records will clearly show what was done and why and the best evidence of that is the contemporaneous notes rather than a statement prepared many months or years later on behalf of a clinician.

Once a patient pursues a claim, practitioners are crucial in clarifying what was said and done in a clinical situation. Without that factual evidence, it is very difficult for the legal teams to accurately estimate the prospects of success of the claim. Clinicians will be asked to provide a statement for use in legal proceedings that covers what was done, why and what is written in the notes. In some cases, clinicians will also be asked what they would have done in a hypothetical situation.

2. CONSENT

The law on capacity and consent to treatment is changing with the introduction of the Mental Capacity Act but this is unlikely to be fully operational until 2007. Meanwhile, before care or treatment is given to a patient, it is crucial that:

- the patient's capacity to consent (or competence) is assessed and that the appropriate action is taken depending on the result of that assessment;
- if the patient has capacity to consent, that they are given the information they need in order to make a decision;
- the patient does consent and that consent is given voluntarily.

If treatment is provided without consent, this may be an assault. It is crucial that all clinicians have a basic understanding of the law of consent and legal advice should be sought where there are areas of uncertainty about how to apply the law to a particular set of clinical circumstances. Assaulting patients gives rise to potential criminal prosecution as well as liability for damages for clinical negligence and the possibility of proceedings before the NMC.

2.1 WHAT IS CONSENT?

Patients can only properly consent to proposed treatment if they have information about it, including information concerning the benefits and risks of the treatment and possible alternative treatments. If the patient is not offered as much information as they reasonably need to make their decision, and in a form they can understand, their consent may not be valid and the treatment they receive may constitute an assault.

2.2 WHAT IS CAPACITY/COMPETENCE?

It is possible for patients to have capacity to make some care/treatment decisions but not others. It is also possible that otherwise competent patients have a particular disorder or phobia which prevents them from believing or weighing up the information that they are given and that this impairs their competence to make a decision about a particular proposal – either permanently or on a temporary basis. Patients can also change their minds and withdraw consent at any time. However, the starting point is that all adults are presumed to be competent unless it is otherwise demonstrated. To have capacity to consent to treatment, patients must be able to comprehend, retain and process the information that they receive about treatment and must be able to understand the consequences of having or not having the treatment.

2.3 PATIENTS WITH CAPACITY

A patient with capacity may not lawfully be given medical treatment without their consent even if they might die or be injured without the treatment. Patient autonomy is paramount where patients have capacity even if the patient's reasons for refusing treatment are not rational (although, if a patient's reasons for refusing treatment appear irrational, this may be an indicator that the treatment's risks and benefits have not properly been explained to them).

Clinical negligence claims relating to consent tend to involve the allegation that there was a failure to warn the patient of a particular risk (such as the risk of cauda equina damage in spinal surgery) which then materialises. Until recently, patients had to satisfy the court that if the missing information had been provided they would have refused the surgery. In a recent case, the patient's evidence was that she could not say if she had been warned of the 1–2% risk of paralysis whether she would have refused to have surgery, but she would have consulted others before proceeding, ie she would not have had surgery that day.

Traditional causation principles (set out earlier) suggest that the patient's claim should have failed because she could not show that the negligence had affected the outcome, ie that she would have refused surgery if properly advised. The House of Lords ruled that it was sufficient for the patient to say that the surgery would not have taken place that day and that the failure to warn the patient denied her the chance to make a fully informed decision. This decision reinforces the importance of providing adequate information to patients and of being able to demonstrate (preferably with reference to patient records that are counter-signed by the patient) that adequate information was provided.

2.4 CHILDREN

Young people aged 16 and 17 are presumed to have the competence to give consent for themselves. Younger children who understand fully what is involved in the proposed procedure can also give consent (although their parents will ideally be involved). In other cases, someone with parental responsibility must give consent on the child's behalf, unless they cannot be reached in an emergency. If a competent child consents to treatment, a parent cannot override that consent. Legally, a parent can consent if a competent child refuses, but this is rare.

2.5 PATIENTS WITHOUT CAPACITY

Under the Mental Capacity Act, it may be possible for someone to consent to treatment on behalf of a person without capacity, and clinicians should keep a careful watch for news of how the act is implemented. At the moment, no one can give consent on behalf of an incompetent adult, and treatment can only be provided if it is in their best interests. 'Best interests' go wider than best medical interests and include factors such as the wishes and beliefs of the patient when competent, their current wishes, their general well-being and their spiritual and religious welfare. People close to the patient may be able to provide information on some of these factors. Where the patient has never been competent, relatives, carers and friends may be best placed to advise on the patient's needs and preferences. If an incompetent patient has clearly indicated in the past, while competent, that they would refuse treatment in certain circumstances (an 'advance refusal'), and those circumstances clearly arise, clinicans must abide by that refusal.

The courts cannot consent on behalf of a patient without capacity but the courts can consider an application for a declaration that a particular treatment is lawful and in the patient's best interests. In cases of doubt, the hospital should seek legal advice on applying to the High Court for such a declaration.

2.6 EMERGENCIES

In an emergency, where consent cannot be obtained, medical treatment may be provided as long as it is limited to what is immediately necessary to save life or avoid significant deterioration in the patient's health, whilst still respecting the terms of any valid advance refusal. Clinicians should tell the patient what has been done, and why, as soon as the patient is sufficiently recovered to understand.

2.7 DEMONSTRATING CONSENT

Consent can be verbal, non-verbal or written. A frequent problem for medico-legal lawyers is that a patient's medical records contain very little information about the consent process. The less information that is available, the more difficult it can be to establish that the consent process was adequate. A bare signature on a consent form does not provide evidence that the patient was given all the appropriate information that they reasonably needed. That information – about the risks and benefits of the procedure and the patient's queries and the response to those queries – should ideally be recorded within the patient's notes as well as any reasons provided by the patient for refusing consent. Ideally, that entry in the records should be counter-signed by the patient.

3. NURSING & MIDWIFERY COUNCIL

The *Nursing & Midwifery Council (NMC)* aims to establish and improve standards of nursing and midwifery care. This section focuses on its work in considering allegations of misconduct or unfitness to practise owing to ill health.

3.1 FITNESS TO PRACTISE

Fitness to practise is defined by the NMC as 'a registrant's suitability to be on the register without restrictions'. The NMC committee considers allegations that a practitioner's fitness to practise is impaired. Allegations may come from a patient, a colleague, a manager or from the police and there is no time limit. Examples of the conduct that has been considered by the committee include:

- sexual, physical or verbal abuse;
- failure to provide adequate care (for managers, this can include failing to maintain an acceptable environment of care);
- failure to keep proper records;
- failure to administer medicines safely;
- deliberately concealing unsafe practice;
- committing criminal offences;
- continued lack of competence despite opportunities to improve;
- a finding by any other health or social care regulator that a registrant's fitness to practise is impaired;
- a fraudulent or incorrect entry in the NMC's register.

Examples of impairment of fitness to practise owing to physical or mental ill health include:

- alcohol or drug dependence;
- untreated serious mental illness.

The NMC guidance emphasises that its aim is to protect the public not to punish practitioners. The standards which the NMC requires of registrants, and which the public is entitled to expect, are set out in the NMC Code of Professional Conduct: Standards for Conduct, Performance and Ethics (the Code). The committee judges conduct and practice on the basis of that Code and by considering registrants against the average standards that it expects of practitioners, not the highest possible level of practice.

3.2 INVESTIGATIVE PROCESS

The NMC has three committees: the Investigating Committee (IC), the Conduct and Competence Committee (CCC) and the Health Committee (HC). Each consists of a number of panels that consider allegations of unfitness to practise. Once a complaint about fitness to practise is received, it is initially forwarded to an (IC) panel which sits in private. The IC considers the available evidence and can either close the case with no further action taken, refer the case to a panel of the CCC or, if related to impairment of fitness to practise for reasons of ill health, refer the case to a panel of the HC.

CCC hearings are generally held in public. The registrant is often represented but the case can proceed even if they are not represented. The CCC panel must decide if the allegation is proven 'beyond reasonable doubt' and will take account of the previous history of the registrant and all the circumstances surrounding the allegations.

Panels of the HC decide whether or not a registrant's fitness to practise is impaired by physical or mental ill health and, if so, whether or not they represent a danger to the public. HC proceedings are generally held in private and attended by the medical examiner who prepared the medical report about the registrant's state of health.

3.3 OPTIONS FOR THE CCC AND HC PANELS

The CCC and HC panels can conclude that the case is not well founded and therefore take no further action. If either panel concludes the case is well founded, it can:

- decide, in all the circumstances, it is not appropriate to take any further action;
- remove the person from the register;
- suspend registration for a specified period not to exceed one year;
- impose conditions of practice for a specified period not to exceed three years;
- issue a caution for a specified period of between one and five years. A caution may be issued only when the facts of the case have been proven and the panel finds the case well founded but there are strong mitigating circumstances.

4. SUMMARY

These are interesting times for nurses with enhanced roles, and the expansion looks set to increase. However, it is in the interests of patients and clinicians alike that expansion is coupled with awareness of the legal implications and, in particular, of the law relating to clinical negligence and consent. It is particularly telling that the NMC Code reminds nurses that they remain responsible for their practice and conduct and that part of responsible practice involves recognising the limits of professional competence and accepting responsibility only for activities that are within that competence.

Part Two
Information Giving and Documentation

6 Communication Skills for Minor Surgery

DEBRA NESTEL

INTRODUCTION

Although knowledge, attitudes and skills relevant to communication are now widely taught in nursing and other healthcare professional curricula (Chant et al. 2002; General Medical Council 2003), the skills necessary for effective patient centred care are often isolated from the real clinical context in which they will be practised. This is especially the case when the communication skills are to be used with other complex technical skills such as ellipse excision and wound closure. This chapter describes an approach to patient centred communication that draws on models of consultations, thereby providing a framework for clinician–patient interactions. The communication skills associated with each stage of a procedural-based encounter are outlined and examples provided of their use in clinical settings. Scenarios are provided as a basis for discussion and reflection. Emphasis is placed on patient assessment, explaining procedures and communicating while performing a procedure. Although skills to communicate effectively with colleagues are also important for safe and effective clinical practice they are beyond the scope of this chapter.

PATIENT CENTRED COMMUNICATION

Before describing the skills necessary for patient centred communication in minor surgery it is helpful to understand theoretical notions of patient centred interactions. Research on 'patient centredness' (Stewart 2001) identifies that patients want care which:

- explores their main reason for the visit, their concerns and need for information;
- provides an integrated understanding of their world – that is, their whole person, emotional needs, and life issues;

Minor Surgical Procedures for Nurses and Allied Healthcare Professionals. Edited by Shirley Martin.
© 2007 John Wiley & Sons Limited

- finds common ground on what the problem is and involves the patient in the decision on how it is to be managed;
- enhances prevention of illness and health promotion;
- enhances the continuing relationship with the clinician.

Research on patient centred interviewing (Putnam and Lipkin 1995) has shown that it provides many benefits for patients, such as:

- improved diagnostic efficiency;
- increase in patient satisfaction;
- increased concordance/adherence with treatments;
- improved recovery rates;
- reduced numbers of symptoms.

Patient centred approaches to care seek to identify, acknowledge and respond to patients' thoughts and feelings throughout entire episodes of illness (or contact with healthcare services). The clinician should seek to understand patients' experience within the broader context of their life and should provide them with an opportunity to understand and participate in their own care to the extent that they want.

PATIENT CENTRED MODEL FOR PROCEDURAL INTERACTIONS

The following model outlines the communication skills necessary for patient centred approaches to care during procedures such a minor surgery. Although clinicians are likely to be familiar with many of these skills, integrating them with technical and other professional skills is challenging. Communication skills are largely generic but their translation to different scenarios can create challenges especially for novices. This section sets out communication skills for the following three key areas of clinician–patient interaction.

1. Patient assessment.
2. Giving information about procedures.
3. Communicating while conducting procedures.

At the end of this chapter models are provided showing ideal communication skills associated with clinical practice. These models are adapted from the undergraduate medical communication programme at Imperial College London and the Calgary-Cambridge Observation Guides (Silverman et al. 2005). They are designed for use in medical practice and focus on interview and consultation skills, rather than assessment, immediately prior to a procedure or during it. They can be used to help you reflect on your clinical practice or can be the basis of an assessment by a colleague who observes you in practice. Role-play and other simulations (professional actors linked with skin pads) can be successfully used in teaching and learning about communication for minor surgery and other procedural skills (Kneebone et al. 2002; Nestel et al. 2003a; Nestel et al. 2003b; Kneebone and Nestel 2005).

1. PATIENT ASSESSMENT

The aim of patient assessments will vary according to your role in minor surgery. They may include making judgments about the suitability of patients for surgery, determining the nature of the surgery, carrying out a pre-procedure assessment after referral, immediate postoperative assessment or assessing the need and providing follow-up care. Not all skills will be used in every interaction. However, whether you are making an initial patient assessment, providing information or conducting a procedure, you must remain sensitive to the patient's well-being. Therefore, the skills described in this part are relevant in all interactions. The skills are divided into four sections – preparation, assessment, relationship building and closing.

Preparing for a patient interaction

Check your own feelings and appearance. Be aware of how you are feeling – rushed, hot, tired, upset, hungry, and if possible deal with these feelings before the interaction. At minimum, be aware that these feelings may influence your behaviour with the patient.

Review the information available on the patient, including any previous interactions with them, and consider what knowledge and equipment you need on this occasion.

Minimise distractions, by turning off mobile telephones and pagers or leaving them with someone who can answer them for you, creating a space in which you can work without interruption.

Initial patient assessment

Generic introductory skills include greeting the patient, giving them your name, and clarifying your role. Use a formal greeting including the patient's name. If the patient is known to you then a less formal greeting may be appropriate.

'Hello, Mr Wilson?'
'Good morning Mr Wilson.'

Touch can have a powerful impact on communication. Shaking hands with patients during your greeting is not essential but is often welcomed. However, some cultures will discourage such touching and you will have to respond to the cues you are given.

Use your full your name and state your role.

> 'My name is Rene Vassar. I am a nurse working with the Minor Surgery Skills Unit.'

Check the patient's comfort. If a patient is uncomfortable they are less likely to be able to concentrate and cooperate. Look at your patient to see if they are uncomfortable, and respond to what you see. Facial expressions are often indicative of a patient's level of comfort. It is helpful to share your observation with your patient, for example, 'You don't seem very comfortable on that chair?', or 'You look as though you are in pain.' Note physical aspects of the environment that contribute to comfort, such as the temperature of the room, draughts, noise, furniture, bedding, etc. Make adjustments where possible.

Assess the patient's ability to communicate with you

Assess whether the patient's ability to communicate with you is compromised by language (not sharing the same language as you), physical disability (hearing, speech or visual impairment) or cultural constraints (cannot make eye contact). Adapt your communication style as much as possible to accommodate these differences. Acknowledge the difficulties as you see them. If you are obtaining consent for a procedure then seeking outside help (interpreter, patient advocate, family member or friend) may be critical.

> 'I only know a little British Sign Language. Would it help to have someone here who knows more?'
> 'We have an interpreting service. I would like to make an appointment to see you again when the interpreter is available.'
> 'I will try to make sure that I am facing you when I speak so that you can see my lips.'
> 'Does it help if I speak more slowly?'
> 'Would it be helpful if I described what I am doing throughout the procedure? That way you will be able to keep track of what I am up to.'

Demonstrate interest and respect

Patients usually respond positively when clinicians are appropriately enthusiastic and non-judgmental, that is, when they are shown genuine interest and respect. This is an important aspect of professional behaviour that sometimes gets lost in busy settings.

Empower the patient to ask questions

Invite patients to ask questions (even though you may not have the answers) and to seek clarification of what you say.

'If anything I say is unclear, please let me know and I will explain.'
'Please feel free to ask me questions.'
'If you have any questions about what I am doing, please ask.'

State the purpose of the interaction

Give the patient a statement of the purpose of the interaction as you see it.

'My role is to assess your need for surgery.'
'I usually see patients who have moles that concern them and make an assessment about their removal.'

Clarify how long the interaction (and procedure) will take

If you have some idea of how long you are going to be with the patient then let them know at the outset.

Use questions effectively

In assessing the patient use open-ended questions initially. These are questions that enable the patient to answer more than 'yes' or 'no.' This helps to ensure that the assessment does not focus too early and that the patient's perspective is presented and valued. Closed-ended questions are useful but not at the beginning of interactions because they tend to narrow the focus of discussion too early. Examples of open-ended questions include:

'Why have you come to the clinic today?'
'How are you feeling?'

In the following example the interviewer moves from open-ended to closed and focused questions.

'You have mentioned the pain in your arm. Can you tell me more about that?' 'Is there anything that seems to bring on the pain?' 'Is there anything that makes it better?'

Avoid leading questions unless they are being used in a summary. These are biased and sometimes judgmental so they may lead the patient to agree with you rather than obtaining accurate information.

'You don't smoke do you?'
'So you've never had stitches before?'

The last question could be used as a means of checking the information you have already gathered which would be acceptable but should not be used as the opening exploratory question. It would be better to ask:

'Have you ever had stitches before?'

Avoid early interruptions

Clinicians have been found to interrupt patients before they have even finished answering the first question of the interaction. It is really important that patients are given some time to talk at the beginning of an interview. This conveys very powerful messages about your level of interest in the patient and your willingness to listen. This listening time may be as brief as a minute but provides the patient with a really important opportunity to express their views. You are likely to gain insight into the patient's understanding of the problem that you otherwise would miss. However, sometimes patients need to be interrupted because the patient is getting increasingly tense, diverging from what is important, or there is a shortage of time or medical urgency associated with a procedure. You need to be able to make appropriate judgments as to when to interrupt. Clear statements of the purpose of the interaction and an indication of the time available can be helpful in managing talkative patients. Non-verbal means of interrupting a patient include the use of clear hand signals or changing body position, adjusting gaze or eye contact.

Identify the patient's ideas, concerns and expectations (ICE)

Although these items are about content rather than skills, they tap into what patients often think are the most important aspects of the interaction, addressing from a patient's perspective the features of patient centred care. Failure to explore and acknowledge the patient's ICE can leave them dissatisfied.

Exploring the patient's ideas might include questions like:

'Many patients have ideas about the cause of their symptoms. Do you?'
'Why do you think you are experiencing these symptoms?'
'Patients often have ideas about possible treatments. What about you?'
'Dr Jennings has recommended that your mole be removed. Do you know what a mole is?'

Understanding the patient's concerns can be gained by asking:

'Do you have any concerns about your operation? Or concerns about anything else?'
'Patients often have worries about cyst removal. Do you?'
'Patients who are having stitches are sometimes anxious about pain or scars. Do these or any other things concern you?'

Assessing the patient's expectations can be achieved by:

'What are you expecting will happen today?'
'What do you think your treatment will be like?'
'Who do you think will be treating you today?'

You do not have to agree with the patient's ideas, allay their concerns or meet their expectations. What is important is that you find out what the baseline position is and work from there. It is usually important to correct misconceptions relating to a patient's problem. There could be key issues in self-care that may not be addressed effectively if the patient has an incorrect understanding of the cause of their problem. Many concerns that patients have can be easily allayed. Others simply need acknowledgment. It is important to be honest with patients about their concerns. Do not offer premature reassurance. Patients may be satisfied with the fact that you cannot meet their expectations. Overt discussion of expectations that cannot be met is more helpful than not raising them at all.

Pick up and respond to verbal and non-verbal cues

Patients sometimes hint at their concerns and it is important that you pick up these leads.

'You mentioned that your brother had a similar experience, can you tell me more about that?'

If patients ask questions, acknowledge the question and try to answer it. If you cannot answer it (because of your own knowledge deficit), then be honest with the patient and offer to find out the answer. Sometimes questions (prognosis and risk) don't have certain answers. Make sure patients understand the uncertainty in your response. Patients can also request information or express worries and fears covertly. Non-verbal behaviours such as facial expressions, eye contact and body positioning and attention can convey important cues to patient's needs. Again, look at patients and respond to what you see. A patient who is distracted may be irritated because you are not focusing on what they want to talk about or may have an overwhelming fear that has not been raised.

Probe sensitively

In some interviews it is important to probe topics very sensitively. These may be topics which many people find sensitive – the death of a family member or taking a sexual history. Acknowledging the difficulty often enables patients to continue.

'I can see this is difficult for you. Do you want to go on . . .?'

Probing sensitively can be assisted by use of the skill 'normalising'. That is, stating the patient's potential fears in a broader context.

'Many patients find it difficult to talk about resuming sex after this sort of surgery, is this difficult for you?'

Clarify patient's terms

Patients sometimes use terms that are colloquial and may require clarification. Do not assume that you know what is meant. Similarly, patients may use medical terms in a way that is different to how you understand them. If you do not know a patient well, then it may be best to check out what they mean when they use terms such as depression or diarrhoea.

Use transition statements

These are statements that link different parts of the interaction together providing structure so you and the patient know what you have covered and what remains.

> 'We have discussed why you have come into the clinic, what I would like to do now is ask you some questions about your health in the past.'
> 'I'd like to start by telling you about the procedure, then I'll prepare the equipment, I'll do the procedure and then tell you what you will have to do to look after your wound at home.'

Make interim summaries

Make brief summaries throughout the interaction in order to check and clarify what you and the patient have exchanged. This also conveys to the patient that you have been listening. It can provide a useful point to change directions in the assessment or explore a topic in greater depth.

> 'I'd like to summarise what you have told me so far . . .'
> 'Just so I can check that I have got this clear, the symptoms first started . . .'
> 'What I have done so far is give you local anaesthetic, I have removed the mole and now I am going to stitch the wound.'

Use silence appropriately

Silence can be very helpful. When people are unwell, highly anxious, or in an unfamiliar place they are often less able to think as quickly as they usually do. Patients often need more time than usual to respond to questions. Silences can be uncomfortable but they can also be used effectively. If you want to work in silence at a particular point in the procedure, then let the patient know.

> 'I'm not going to talk for a few minutes because I need to really concentrate while I clean your wound.'
> 'I just want to make notes on the information you have given me so far.'

Building the relationship

Throughout each stage it is important to use communication skills to establish and maintain your relationship with the patient. The following skills overlap with many of those outlined above but are listed again because of their importance in building and maintaining relationships with patients.

Use non-verbal communication effectively

Non-verbal communication such as eye contact, body posture, gestures, facial expressions and touch are incredibly powerful. Having made eye contact with the patient when first meeting, maintaining this appropriately throughout the interaction will depend in part on the patient's reaction to you. In principle, non-verbal communication that conveys to the patient that they are the focus of your attention is vital. Although analysis of specific behaviours is helpful when learning about communication, patients usually respond to the overall impact of these behaviours. Attention to the arrangement of physical space for interviewing can influence the communication, for example sitting adjacent rather than opposite to patients, sitting at the same level. Personal space also needs to be considered – neither too close nor too far. Touch may be appropriate in a consultation – it can convey reassurance, identify specific body parts, and it forms part of clinical examinations and many procedures. However, you will need to be guided by patients' responses because cultural factors constrain the appropriateness of touch.

Use verbal communication effectively

Verbal communication consists of the content of your speech as well as paralinguistic characteristics. These include the clarity, pace, tone and volume of your voice that together can be used to add power to the content of your message. Think about the structure of the interaction and try to be logical, although it is important to be flexible in order to respond to patients' needs.

Use clear and simple terms to describe what you are doing. This is not patronising. If the purpose of information exchange is to be effective then clarity and simplicity are crucial. Jargon and medical terms need to be explained. Think about creative ways in which jargon can be explained. Pictures, diagrams, models, and body parts can be helpful. In minor surgery commonly used terms that may not be understood by patients include biopsy, sutures, and LA. Use them but explain them first.

Other terms often used by clinicians also convey interesting messages to the patient. The term 'little' is frequently used to describe incisions, injections, biopsies, blood, or dressings, which to the patient's way of thinking may not be 'little' at all. The term seems to be used to help clinicians feel more comfortable about what they are doing to the patient.

Use active listening

Active listening can be demonstrated verbally by staying with the patient's topic, using the patient's words, reflecting statements back to the patient and making summaries. Non-verbal skills used in active listening include using eye contact, nodding, body posture, setting up your procedure trolley facing the patient, avoiding note taking or using the computer while the patient is talking, and sitting or standing still while talking about important topics.

Make empathic statements

Empathy is identifying what a patient is feeling, and communicating this understanding. After the patient has expressed a feeling, an empathic statement can make a personal connection with the patient. Emotions are also expressed non-verbally.

'Yes, I can see you are in pain.'
'That must have been very difficult managing all those years.'
'I can tell from what you are saying that it was a distressing time for you.'
'I hear what you are saying about your depression. It can be extremely difficult.'
'You still seem worried.'
'It is okay to be upset.'

Show warmth

Showing warmth combines several verbal and non-verbal skills. Warmth refers to your acceptance of the patient. This does not mean that you agree or support the patient's views but it conveys respect. This can be achieved by listening, by staying with the patient's topic, by acknowledging that you have understood what they are saying, by your body position, facial expressions, eye contact, silence and the tone and volume of your voice.

Although you will almost certainly hold many strong views about a whole range of subjects, in clinical care it is important that those views are only shared appropriately, if at all. You will be confronted by patients who may trigger various feelings in you that in non-clinical life might cause you to make judgments about them. People who hold strong religious beliefs (or none at all), who smoke, gamble, are obese (or have other eating disorders), drink and drive, have alcohol problems, are paedophiles, murderers, rapists, etc. As a professional you are expected not to let your judgments about beliefs and character get in the way of the care you provide.

Closing the interaction

Provide an end summary

Before finishing the interview it is valuable to make a summary. It means that you can check with the patient the accuracy of the information exchanged as well as leave the patient with a sense of what you both thought important. Lasting impressions are just as important as first impressions. An end summary also signals to the patient that you are about to finish. If you have just finished a procedure then it is helpful to state precisely what you have done. Patients are sometimes anxious while you are conducting procedures and so are less able to remember what you have told them.

'I'd like to summarise what we have discussed.'
'I'm going to tell you what I have just done and what is going to happen next.'

Discuss an action plan

State what will happen next. Be explicit in relation to what you will do and what the patient needs to do, when and how.

Check for further questions

Sometimes patients wait until the last moment to ask key questions, especially if you have not provided them with an opportunity to do so earlier or patients may not feel comfortable asking for or sharing information earlier. Therefore, it is helpful to ask if the patient has any further queries or comments immediately before the end of the interview. Again, patients are assimilating information throughout the interaction and your summary might have triggered an area of discussion they would like to pursue. Also, check if the patient has any new worries or concerns. New concerns may have emerged during the interview.

'When we first started talking you mentioned you were worried about the timing of the operation. Now that we have clarified that, I was wondering if you had any other concerns.'

2. GIVING INFORMATION ABOUT PROCEDURES

Giving information to patients is fundamental to most clinical roles. Although most clinicians develop extensive knowledge of procedures and operations, it is likely that this is solely from their specialist perspective. This is essential for them to function effectively with other healthcare professionals but patients usually require information about procedures and operations that is from a different perspective. Clinicians need to assess each patient's need for information and to address these needs in a way that patients will understand and remember. Patients usually want answers to the questions listed in Table 6.1. There are important principles to be followed when giving information that relate to teaching and learning in any setting, so that understanding and recall can be helped. Table 6.2 provides a general model for patient centred assessment, while Table 6.3 is a model for explaining about procedures.

Table 6.1 Questions patients often want answers to in relation to procedures or tests

What is it (test/procedure/operation)?
How painful it will be?
Will I be awake?
What can go wrong?
What are the chances of something going wrong?
When will it take place?
Where will it happen?
What preparation is necessary?
How long will the procedure/test last?
Will I have a scar?
Who else will be present?
What happens afterwards?
What are possible side/after effects?
When will the result be available?
Who will give the result?
Can I go home afterwards?

Table 6.2 Model for patient centred assessment of patients in minor surgery

	Not done	Needs development	Done well	N/A
Preparing for the interaction				
1 Checks own feelings and appearance				
2 Reviews patient information and resources				
3 Minimises distractions				
Commencing the interaction				
4 Makes generic introduction (greeting, states name, role, uses patient's name, checks patient comfort, assesses patient ability to communicate, demonstrates interest and respect, empowers the patient to ask questions)				

Table 6.2 *Continued*

	Not done	Needs development	Done well	N/A
5 Makes specific introduction (states purpose of interaction, clarifies how long the interaction will take)				

Assessing the patient

	Not done	Needs development	Done well	N/A
6 Uses questions effectively (open-ended initially, moves to closed-ended, avoids leading questions)				
7 Avoids early interruptions				
8 Identifies patient's ideas, concerns and expectations				
9 Picks up and responds to patient's verbal cues (questions, deviations from topic, requests for information, worries)				
10 Picks up and responds to patient's non-verbal cues (facial expression, silence, anxiety, lack of eye contact, fidgeting)				
11 Probes sensitively				
12 Clarifies patient's terms				
13 Uses transition statements				
14 Makes interim summaries				
15 Uses silence effectively				

Building the relationship

	Not done	Needs development	Done well	N/A
16 Uses non-verbal communication effectively(eye contact, body language, touch, facial expressions, silence)				
17 Uses verbal communication effectively (clear and audible speech, logical, avoids jargon, language is understandable, explains medical terms)				
18 Uses active listening (verbal – staying with patient's topic, using patient's words, reflection; non-verbal – body posture, gestures, eye contact, facial expressions, nodding, stillness)				
19 Makes empathic statements ('I can see you are worried', 'You seem anxious')				
20 Shows warmth (respectful, non-judgmental, vocal qualities, eye contact)				

Closing the interaction

	Not done	Needs development	Done well	N/A
21 Provides an end summary				
22 Discusses an action plan				
23 Checks for further information required				
24 Checks if the patient has any new worries or concerns				

Table 6.3 Model for patient centred information giving about procedures

	Not done	Needs development	Done well	N/A
Giving information about procedures				
1 General description of the procedure (purpose, what happens, rationale)				
2 Specific information (is it painful, how long it takes, who does it, risks, side effects, sedation, results available)				
3 Provides accurate information				
4 Uses skills to aid understanding and recall (organised, logical, explicit categorisation, repetition, emphasis, specific versus general information, summaries)				
5 Gives information within patient's framework of understanding (relates to earlier questions, concerns, worries, ideas, expectations)				

Starting point

Find the right level at which to pitch the information by establishing what the patient already knows.

'What have you been told so far?'
'What have you been told about the procedure?'
'Have you ever had stitches before?'
'What do you know about the removal of cysts?'

Information needs

Find out what the patient wants to know and if specific information has a priority. This needs to be balanced with what you are obliged to tell the patient.

'Is there anything else you would like to know about?'
'There is certain information I am obliged to give you but I was wondering if there was anything you especially wanted to know?'

Primacy and recency effect

People remember what they hear first and last. This is referred to as the primacy and recency effect. If information is important place it at the beginning or the end of the interaction.

Emphasis

If you have information that is really important then use emphasis by stating precisely that, and use vocal characteristics to reinforce the message.

'It is really important that you try to remember about the allergic reaction.'

'This is the most important thing to remember today. If you feel pain, see redness in the wound, have a fever or see anything coming out of the wound, then you must return to the clinic immediately.'

Repetition

We are more likely to remember things that are repeated. As well as using emphasis, repeat important information.

Explicit categorisation

People remember information in 'chunks' so breaking the information into meaningful categories and then making these explicit can be helpful in delivering information so that it is understood and remembered.

'What I can do is tell you what will happen before the procedure, during it and then afterwards. Would this be helpful?'

'First, I will tell you what happens before the procedure. Second, I will tell you what happens during the procedure. Third, and finally, I will tell you what happens afterwards. Is that okay?'

'When you leave the hospital it is important to consider three things: first, caring for your wound; second, taking your medicine; third, coming back for your results.'

Specific versus general information

Information which is personalised and so directly related to the patient's experience is more likely to be understood and therefore remembered. This can only be done if you have explored the patient's ideas, concerns and expectations and established a relationship with them. This can be achieved in relatively brief interactions if the skills described in patient assessment are implemented.

'From what you have said about your work schedule, I suspect it might be best to have a morning appointment.'

'Your concern about your weight is something we can act on. Rather than focus on this today, it might be best to deal with the surgery first and then as part of your follow-up care put you in touch with the dietitian who is very experienced in working with patients with your condition.'

Summaries

By consolidating information a summary can help patients to understand and remember what you have told them.

> 'I'd like to summarise what we have discussed so far. Before I start the procedure, I need to have your written consent. Then, I will take you to the procedure room where I will arrange the equipment and then we can get started. This part should take just a few minutes.'

3. COMMUNICATING WHILE CONDUCTING PROCEDURES

We have considered the skills needed to communicate with patients during assessment and when providing them with information. We now deal with the communication skills that are important during procedures. Table 6.4 sets these out in summary.

Developing patient centred communication skills

- To what extent do you allow patients to express their concerns? What communication skills do you use to facilitate this? How do you know a patient has expressed their major concern/s?
- Do you 'routinely' ask patients if they have any specific requests? Make a list of patients' specific requests – perhaps the last five patients you have seen. Are there any requests that surprise you? Why is it important that you identify specific requests from patients?
- Do you ask patients for their views about why they are ill? How do you ask? Record a patient's explanation for symptoms that differed to your own view. What are 'feelings'? What are 'thoughts'? Why is it important that clinicians understand the difference between these? Do you ask patients about their feelings? How do you ask?

Table 6.4 Model for patient centred communication during procedures

	Not done	Needs development	Done well	N/A
Communicating while operating				
1 Integrates communication with technical skills				
2 Offers to describe what is happening throughout procedure				
3 Gives patient cues to interrupt				
4 Offers supportive verbal communication				
5 Demonstrates awareness of patient's comfort throughout procedure				

- Do you always 'hear' patients' answers to your questions?
- To what extent do you think the information you provide to patients is centred on their needs? To what extent do you give all patients the same information about procedures? When interacting with patients, what proportion of time do you spend giving information? Do you think you overestimate the time you spend giving information to patients?
- What skills do you think are most important for giving information to patients?
- To what extent do you include patients in decisions about their treatment? To what extent do you discuss options? How do you assess a patient's willingness to participate in their treatment? Record an example of a patient whom you have successfully included in their treatment plan.

Integrate communication and technical skills

It is apparent that inexperienced clinicians tend to stop 'communicating' once the procedure has started. Although talking may take place it is often 'disconnected'. That is, clinicians may ignore important cues from the patient because they are over-focused on their technical task. Self-awareness is important. It may be helpful to let patients know that you are going to work in silence at particular points in the procedure. A poignant example of this disconnection is the clinician who during a procedure to remove a mole responded to the patient who had just expressed his fear of melanoma following his brother's death from the disease with the statement – 'I'm just going to wash my hands.' The clinician was so focused on preparing for the procedure that there was a failure to acknowledge this important fear and the patient's grief. This changed the quality of the relationship from the patient's perspective, although the clinician continued in ignorance. On reviewing videotaped footage of the encounter the clinician could not believe what she had done.

Offer to describe what is happening

Sometimes clinicians give a running narrative of what they are doing. Although some patients find this helpful, it is not appropriate for all patients so offer to keep the patient informed of your actions rather than assuming the patient wants to hear.

> 'Some patients like me to describe exactly what I am doing in the procedure. Would you like this?'

If there is a problem during the procedure, give the patient brief and honest information about what is happening.

> 'I am having trouble closing the wound. I'd like to seek advice from my colleague. Please stay as you are. It is important that you do not touch the wound or your drape. I will just be a couple of minutes.'

Give the patient cues to interrupt

If patients are likely to experience discomfort during the procedure then be explicit about what this might be, how the patient might cope (look away, breath deeply) and how the patient can convey that their discomfort is intolerable. If you will not be able to see the patient's facial expressions, let them know that they should tell you if they want you to stop.

Offer verbal encouragement

Reporting your progress during the procedure can provide support to patients in coping with discomfort.

> 'I am about halfway through now. The worst part is over as far as pain goes. Do you think you can go on?'
> 'Good. You are doing really well. Everything is progressing as I would expect.'

Demonstrate awareness of patient's comfort throughout the procedure

It is crucial to monitor the patient's feelings and physical status throughout the procedure. This involves verbal and non-verbal skills – looking, listening and responding.

Closing

Closing is often done less effectively than other parts of the interaction – possibly in an effort to move on to the next patient having completed the technical task. However, this is potentially a crucial phase for the patient as it could include education and other self-care information. The effectiveness of time taken to explain what has been done, what happens next and checks that the patient has understood can be greatly dimished if it is combined with tidying up and other activity. Try to take a minute to stop and focus on the patient in the same way that you did when you started the interaction.

Reflecting on patient centred communication

Communication is relevant to everything we do in clinical settings and it can be challenging to stop and reflect on what we actually do and to think about how others see us, but undertaking this is extremely worth while. Table 6.1 lists a series of questions designed to help you reflect on how you communicate with patients. There are no correct answers. Personal reflections are a starting point for taking a fresh look at your clinical communication. It is important to remember that what you think you do in practice is not always what you actually do. Seeking feedback from colleagues and patients as well as making the time to review your interactions on videotape are powerful learning experiences.

Discussion that reflect on patient centred communication in minor surgery

Below are two scenarios that focus on communication in minor surgery. These are designed for discussion to help you apply the theoretical concepts outlined in this chapter to real clinical situations. Again, there are no correct answers although some points will be more important than others (Nestel et al. 2003c).

Scenario 1

You have just made an ellipse excision to remove a lesion from your patient's arm. She becomes very tearful. What might you do in this situation?

Possible discussion points.

- Importance of careful observation (looking at and listening to patients throughout procedures, checking whether their non-verbal and verbal communication is synchronous).
- Role of empathic statements ('I can see you're distressed but I am not sure why. Can I do anything to help you?').
- Making assumptions about the cause of the emotion (it could be any number of reasons, some may be more obvious than others – avoid making assumptions).
- Reassurance can only be offered after the source of the emotion is identified.
- Options for the clinician and patient (Do you continue? Do you ask a colleague to close the wound? Do you give the patient time to settle down?).
- Issues around maintaining asepsis (Do you touch the patient? Gloves on or off?).

Scenario 2

You have just successfully completed an ellipse excision and closed the wound after removal of a lesion. The patient asks you what happens next. What might you do?

Possible discussion points.

- Find out what the patient wants to know. What are their priorities? What are your priorities? What do you deal with first?
- What skills do you use to ensure understanding?
- Ask for concerns.
- Ask for questions.
- What questions might the patient have? (What happens to the tissue that was removed? How do I care for my wound? What should I do about pain? Can I get the wound wet? Does the dressing need to be changed? What happens to the stitches? Will I see a doctor again?)

Summary

In this chapter models for communication have been outlined that reflect patient centred approaches to caring for patients undergoing minor surgery. The models describe different aspects of clinician–patient interactions. Not all the communication skills will be used in every interaction. Clinicians will need to select the skills that are relevant to the context in which they are working and, most importantly, appropriate to the individual patient in front of them. Clinician–patient communication is a critical factor in clinical safety. Taking time to reflect on and develop your clinical communication skills is an important component of professional behaviour.

REFERENCES

Chant S, Jenkinson T, Randle J, Russell G (2002) Communication skills: some problems in nursing education. *Journal of Clinical Nursing* **11**, 12–21.

General Medical Council (2003) *Tomorrow's Doctors: Recommendations on Undergraduate Medical Education*. London: GMC.

Kneebone RL, Kidd J, Nestel D, Asvall S, Paraskeva P, Darzi A (2002) An innovative model for teaching and learning clinical procedures. *Medical Education* **36** (7), 628–634.

Kneebone RL, Nestel D (2005) Learning clinical skills – the place of simulation. *Clinical Teacher* **2**, 86–90.

Nestel D, Kneebone RL, Kidd J (2003a) Teaching and learning about skills in minor surgery – an innovative course for nurses. *Journal of Clinical Nursing* **12** (2), 291–296.

Nestel D, Kneebone R, Taylor P (2003b) Communication for gastrointestinal endoscopy: Experiences of a course for nurse practitioners. *Gastrointestinal Nursing* **1** (8), 18–25.

Nestel D, Kneebone R, Martin S (2003c) Interprofessional learning: discussion groups in a minor surgery course for nurses. *Nursing Education in Practice* **3**, 1–8. ISSN 1471-5953.

Putnam S, Lipkin M (1995) The patient centred interview: research support. In: Lipkin M, Putnam S, Lazare A. *The Medical Interview: Clinical Care, Education and Research.* Ann-Arbour: Springer-Verlag.

Silverman J, Kurtz S, Draper J (2005) *Skills for Communicating with Patients.* (2nd edn). Oxford: Radcliffe Medical Press.

Stewart M (2001) Towards a global definition of patient centred care. *British Medical Journal*, **322**, 444–445.

7 Preoperative Assessment

ANURAG PATEL AND SANJAY PURKAYASTHA

More than 3 million operative procedures are carried out each year within the NHS. It is fundamental that there are optimally functioning processes to ensure that a patient receives excellent care and ultimately a safe and successful intervention/procedure.

The focus of this chapter is preoperative assessment, an important part of your patient's care. Why is there need for assessing patients preoperatively? This can largely be answered by asking three further questions.

- Has the patient been listed for the correct procedure?
- Does the patient still require the procedure?
- What can be done to ensure that the patient can safely be given a general anaesthetic (GA) and undergo surgical procedure?

We will expand later on these questions but it is important that answers are sought and addressed early and not on the day of the procedure. This optimises patient fitness prior to elective surgery and minimises the risk of last-minute cancellations. (The role of preoperative assessment in reducing the incidence of cancellations on the day of surgery, J Cotton, Birmingham Women's Hospital, Abstract from The Preoperative Association First National Conference, Nottingham, 18–19 Oct 2004.) Preoperative assessment can maximise theatre utilisation and therefore reduce waiting lists. (How preoperative assessment has reduced DNAs and cancellations on the day of operation, S Roberts, Salford Royals Hospitals NHS Trust, Abstract from The Preoperative Association First National Conference, Nottingham, 18–19 Oct 2004.)

Preoperative assessment is a field in its own right and it is rapidly evolving in the UK. The first national conference of the Preoperative Association was held in October 2004 (www.pre-op.org). NICE has published a useful guide to 'the use of routine preoperative tests in elective surgery' (Preoperative Tests: The Use of Preoperative Tests in Elective Surgery. NICE June 2003). The use and development of preoperative assessment questionnaires is spreading throughout Trusts but a national protocol is needed and this is currently being addressed by the Preoperative Association.

Minor Surgical Procedures for Nurses and Allied Healthcare Professionals. Edited by Shirley Martin.
© 2007 John Wiley & Sons Limited

The use of integrated care pathways (ICPs) for certain procedures within specialties should not detract from seeking answers to the three fundamental questions, thereby ensuring thorough preoperative assessment of your patient. Examples of ICPs in medical literature include: 'ICP for carotid endarterectomy' (*British Journal of Nursing* (2002, Sept.); and 'The development of a patient-centred care pathway for total abdominal hysterectomy' (*Nursing Standards* (2003, Oct.). It is important to be familiar with which ICPs are currently being used in your Trust and to ensure that a thorough preoperative assessment forms part of these pathways.

ADDRESSING THE THREE FUNDAMENTAL QUESTIONS

HAS THE PATIENT BEEN LISTED FOR THE CORRECT PROCEDURE?

Patient history and examination.

Correspondence, eg outpatient letter indicating reasons for listing patient for surgical procedure.

DOES THE PATIENT STILL REQUIRE THE PROCEDURE?

Does correspondence match patient's current history and examination? If NO – seek help. If YES – continue to Question 3.

WHAT CAN BE DONE TO ENSURE THAT THE PATIENT CAN SAFELY BE GIVEN A GENERAL ANAESTHETIC (GA) AND UNDERGO SURGICAL PROCEDURE?

This last question forms the basis for patient assessment preoperatively and answers to the following categories will highlight potential conditions and problems which need addressing.

Medical history

Medical

Cardiovascular.
Any new symptoms from systemic enquiry.
Heart failure – follow New York Heart Association classification (see Appendix 7.1).
IHD – follow Canadian classification of mild and severe angina (see Appendix 7.2).
Valvular defect/prosthesis.

Previous MI.
Thromboembolism.
Respiratory.
TB, COPD, Asthma.
Endocrine.
Diabetes.
Pituitary, thyroid, pancreatic, adrenal disorders.
Neurological.
Mobility issues.
Previous or recent TIAs or CVAs.
Epilepsy.
Gastrointestinal/Urinary Systems.
Surgery.
Anaesthetics.

Allergies and present medications

Particular attention must be drawn to patients taking the following.

Anticoagulants/antiplatelet aggregation.
Cardiovascular medication.
Respiratory medication.
Antiepileptic medication.
Diabetic medication.

Social history

Alcohol intake.
Smoking (quantity and duration, including ex-smokers).
Social support/environment.
Functional/mobility.

Family history

General anaesthetic.
Surgical.
Medical.

INVESTIGATIONS

Information gathered from the above questions will enable you to tailor the investigations for your patient depending on the type of surgical procedure envisaged. Before ordering investigations one must always ask why your patient needs them. NICE has provided the following invaluable guidelines to the advantages of requesting a preoperative investigation.

- To provide information that may confirm or question the correctness of the current course of clinical management.
- To be able to use this information to reduce the possible harm or increase the benefit to patients by altering their clinical management if necessary.
- To be able to use this information to help assess the risk to the patient and to open the possibility of discussing potential risks with the patient.
- To more easily predict postoperative complications.
- To establish baseline measurements for later reference.
- To provide opportunistic screening that is unrelated to surgery.

However, it is worth pointing out that the NHS Health Technology Assessment review of preoperative assessment concluded that 'a policy of pre operative testing in apparently healthy individuals is likely to lead to little, if any, benefit (HTA 1997; 1(12), i–iv).

We give below guides from two major sources to carrying out various investigations based on guidelines from various respected bodies in each of the specialties. We see this guide as necessary due to the lack of adequate randomising controlled trials comparing the outcomes of patients who, preoperatively, had routine investigations compared with those who had indicated preoperative investigations.

ASA guidelines

The American Society of Anesthesiologists' (ASA) practice advisory for preanaesthesia evaluation provides useful evidence-based guidelines for preoperative tests (Practice Advisory for Preanesthesia Evaluation. A report by the ASA Task Force on Preanesthesia Evaluation, 15 October 2003. [http://www.asahq.org/publicationsAndServices/preeval.pdf]).

ECG

Indicated for patients with known cardiovascular risk factors or for patients with risk factors identified in the course of a preanaesthesia evaluation. The ASA taskforce recognises that age alone may not be an indication for ECG.

CXR

The ASA provides the following clinical characteristics for consideration: smoking, recent upper respiratory infection, COPD and cardiac disease. It should be noted that the ASA states that 'the task force does not believe that the extremes of age, smoking, stable COPD, stable cardiac disease, or resolved upper respiratory infection should be considered as unequivocal indications for CXR'.

Hb

Should not be carried out routinely and should only be considered in patients with liver disorders, previous/current anaemia, previous history of bleeding or other haematological disorders. The decision should also take into account the invasiveness of the procedure.

Coagulation studies

Although the ASA task force provides no evidence-based guidelines in this area, they state that the following clinical characteristics should be considered: renal dysfunction, liver dysfunction, bleeding disorders, type and invasiveness of procedure.

Biochemical tests

Consider clinical characteristics such as use of certain medical therapies, use of perioperative therapies, risk of renal or liver dysfunction, and endocrine disorders.

Urinanalysis

Presence of UTI symptoms or dependent on specific procedures, eg urological.

Pregnancy testing

Should be offered to women of child bearing age and performed for those for whom the outcome will alter the patient's management.

NICE preoperative tests guidelines

(http:/www.nice.org.uk/catasp?c+56818).

ECG

There is value in ECG for increasing age and ASA grade but no definitive guideline. This is due to the lack of evidence comparing health outcomes for individuals who did and did not undergo a preoperative ECG.

CXR

NICE emphasises that there is no direct evidence for or against carrying out a preoperative CXR but there may be value in this investigation with a patient's increasing age or ASA grade.

Hb

Implies value with increasing age but no definitive guidelines due to the lack of evidence, again with regard to outcome measurement in individuals with and without preoperative FBC assessment.

Coagulation studies

Although evidence infers value in performing this test with increasing comorbidity, ie increasing ASA grade, there is no direct evidence that such a test will or will not improve health outcomes.

Biochemical tests

No evidence suggests that abnormalities increase with age or comorbidities. Therefore no guideline or attributable value is inferred.

Urinanalysis

There may be value with increasing age and comorbidity, ie increasing ASA grade, but no direct evidence available to infer improved health outcomes.

Pregnancy testing

No evidence to compare health outcome measures with and without pre-operative testing but there is evidence that positive pregnancy tests led to a decision to cancel or postpone procedure, or loss of foetus when surgery went ahead despite positive result.

Pulmonary function tests

No direct evidence.

ABGs

No sufficient evidence.

Appendix 7.1

New York Heart Association Classification

Class I – no undue symptoms during ordinary activity, no limitation of physical activity.

Class II – slight limitation of physical activity, comfortable at rest.

Class III – marked limitation of physical activity, comfortable at rest.

Class IV – no physical activity possible without discomfort, symptoms at rest.

Class I&II = compensated.

Class III&IV = decompensated.

Source: The Criteria Committee of the New York Heart Association (1994) Nomenclature and Criteria for Diagnosis of Diseases of the Heart and Great Vessels. (9th edn). Boston: Little Brown & Co. www.americanheart. org/presenter.jhtml?identifier=1712 (accessed 12/11/04).

Appendix 7.2

Canadian Classification of Mild and Severe Angina

Class I – angina on strenuous activity only.

Class II – slight limitation of ordinary activity (eg >1 flight of stairs).

Class III – marked limitation of ordinary activity (eg <1 flight of stairs, walking level).

Class IV – angina at rest.

Class I&II = mild.

Class III &IV = severe.

Source: Campeau L. (1976) Grading of angina pectoris [letter] *Circulation.* **54**, 522–523.

Appendix 7.3

ASA Physical Status Classification System

Grade I – normal healthy patient.

Grade II – mild systemic disease.

Grade III – severe systemic disease.

Grade IV – severe systemic disease that is a constant threat to life.

Grade V – moribund where patient is not expected to survive without operation.

Grade VI – formally declared as brain dead where organs are removed for donor purposes.

Source: www.asahq.org/clinical/physicalstatus.htm (accessed 12/11/04).

Appendix 7.4

Severity of Surgery Grades (NICE)

Grade I – eg diagnostic endoscopy/laparoscopy, breast biopsy.

Grade II – eg inguinal hernia, varicose veins, adenotonsillectomy, knee arthroscopy.

Grade III – eg total abdominal hysterectomy, lumber discectomy, TURP, thyroidectomy.

Grade IV – eg total joint replacement, arterial reconstruction, colonic resection, radical neck dissection.

Source: www.pre-op.org/docs/utilities/guidelines%20_for_preoperative_ testing.pdf (accessed 12/11/04).

Appendix 7.5

Dyspnoea Scale

Grade I – no dyspnoea while walking on the level at normal pace.

Grade II – short of breath when hurrying or walking up a slight hill. Not affected by any distance provided 'I take my time'.

Grade III – walks slower than contemporaries on level ground because of breathlessness. Limited by specific distance and has to stop for breath when walking at own pace.

Grade IV – limited by mild exertion, eg needing to stop and rest 'from going from kitchen to bathroom'.

Source: adapted from Fletcher CM, Elmes PC, Fairbairn MB et al. (1959) The significance of respiratory symptoms and the diagnosis of chronic bronchitis in a working population. *BMJ* 2:57–66 and Roizen's classification.

8 Perioperative Management, Consent and Follow-up

JENNIFER SIMPSON

INTRODUCTION

As nurses take on more autonomous and specialised roles and expand the scope of their practice it is vital that they 'get it right', ensuring that a profession under growing scrutiny demonstrates the required high level of competence (Oxtoby 2005). Traditionally, information on specific procedures and their risks and benefits has been solely within the domain of the medical profession. However, with the publication and implementation of measures such as the Scope of Professional Practice (UKCC 1992), the Calman Report (with the subsequent reduction in junior doctors' hours), the Ten Key Roles for Nurses and Midwives and the new ways of working initiatives, nurses have been enabled to take on some of the tasks previously carried out by the medical profession.

Before undertaking minor surgical procedures, all healthcare professionals need to equip themselves with the appropriate skills, so that they can perform these procedures as competently and as safely as possible. This requires both receiving and imparting a variety of verbal and written information, and the ability to produce it if necessary.

The sharing of information by providing health education to patients undergoing any form of surgery is an essential role for the healthcare professional. When seeking written consent the patient should be given sufficient information, in plain understandable language, as early as possible, to allow them sufficient time to make a decision (NHSLA 2004).

Tingle (1998) highlighted some of the implications for nurses who are taking on tasks such as minor surgery, suggesting that appropriate training is advisable and that any such knowledge needs to be maintained and updated regularly. Any nurse undertaking these procedures should be assessed as being competent to perform the role at the level of the medical practitioner.

Lee Gledhill (2005), a barrister specialising in medical law, maintains that 'nurses can only seek valid consent or obtain valid consent if they are trained

Minor Surgical Procedures for Nurses and Allied Healthcare Professionals. Edited by Shirley Martin.
© 2007 John Wiley & Sons Limited

in all aspects of that, and also only if they know the area of clinical practice well'. Failure to adhere to proper consent procedures, for example, can result in criminal prosecution for assault or neglect, a civil law suit or referral to the Nursing and Midwifery Council (NMC) for professional misconduct (Oxtoby 2005) if the health professional is a nurse. The NMC provides specific guidance on the issue of consent in clause 3 of the NMC Code of Professional Conduct (2004).

The Department of Health (DH) has also produced various guidelines to assist with the consent process by highlighting the necessity for the health professional to provide appropriate information about the patient's condition and the possible risks and benefits (including the risks/benefits of doing nothing (DH 2003). The Medical Protection Society, which provides advice for members of the General Medical Council, also provides essential guidance on consent to medical students, GPs and consultants. This guidance is equally relevant to non-medically trained professionals such as Surgical Care Practitioners (SCPs) and other allied health professionals, who may be expanding their roles.

A recent decision by the House of Lords in the case of *Chester* v. *Afshar*, has significantly extended clinicians' liabilities in cases where less than full consent is obtained. This decision has serious implications for practitioners in the NHS as well as in private practice. Failure to obtain adequate consent now overrides any argument that such failure did not cause an adverse outcome.

This chapter will discuss the importance of providing information to the patient and the need to develop appropriate communication skills when obtaining consent for minor surgical procedures. There are many issues surrounding the consent process which cannot all be covered here and it is therefore suggested that the reader reinforces this information from the list of essential reading given at the end of the chapter.

THE CONSENT PROCESS

PATIENT INFORMATION

THE BENEFITS

Good patient information is important as it can serve several vital functions. The Department of Health (2003) maintains that it provides the following benefits.

- Patients are given confidence, improving their experience.
- Patients are reminded of the main points discussed.
- Enables informed decisions to be made, with time to absorb and reflect on the information.
- Ensures patients arrive on time for appointments.
- Ensures involvement of patients and their carers.
- Helps to reduce patient anxieties.

PRESENTATION

All patient information should be:

- **clear** – so it can be understood;
- **straightforward** – using few words and less medical jargon;
- **accessible** – available to as many people as possible, given at the right time at the right place;
- **up to date** – evidenced based and reviewed regularly;
- **respectful** – sensitive to the cultural needs of all people;
- **cost effective** – printed material may be better than photocopies in terms of both cost and quality.

Information is an important part in the patient journey and is a key element in the overall quality of the patient's experience (DH 2003).

A commitment in the NHS Plan (DH 2000) and part of the service's recommendations in the Kennedy Report is the improving and monitoring of information to patients. To achieve this the DH has developed a toolkit for producing patient information (2003) which includes essential guidance on how to produce written information for patients, together with a series of templates. The Clinical Negligence Schemes for Trusts (CNST 2005) also provides guidance in relation to providing appropriate information and gaining informed consent. The scheme advises that every Trust should have in place a procedure for the timing and method of giving information to the patient, and which is documented on the consent form. This procedure needs to take account of the fact that the needs of day patients differ from those of inpatients.

A well-informed patient minimises the risks. Once a decision to have a particular treatment/investigation has been made, patients need information about what will happen, where to go, how long they will be expected to stay in hospital, how they will feel afterwards and what to look for in terms of complications, etc. In the short time they spend in hospital, every contact between a patient and health professional should be used as an opportunity for receiving and giving information (Sutherland 1996.)

Communication with the patient is essential and should begin at initial referral. Most patients would have most likely had an initial assessment and diagnosis made by a doctor, whether a GP or hospital consultant who has ultimate responsibility for the care of that patient. Depending upon the type of service being offered, for example a one stop minor surgery service, the patient should receive written information regarding the date surgery will be carried out, where to attend and any preoperative instructions (see Figure 8.1).

This is an ideal opportunity to provide details about local anaesthesia used to suppress any pain during the procedure, and what they can expect in terms of how long the procedure will take, postoperative pain relief, wound care advice and so on, providing specific information on the intended procedure if this is available. If patients arrive unprepared and ignorant about what is about to happen to them it is up to the health professional to ensure they understand and also to help relieve any anxiety or concerns they may have (see Figure 8.2).

COMMUNICATION SKILLS

On the day of intended surgery it is important to establish a rapport with the patient to elicit appropriate information from them and to reinforce the information they have been given. This can be achieved by the development of good communication skills.

The initial interview with the patient should include an assessment of their ability to comprehend what is being said. The Medical Protection Society (2003) suggest that in order to give consent an adult individual must be 'competent' and should be able to:

- understand information that has been presented to them;
- believe the information they have been given;
- retain it long enough to make a decision.

By utilising simple, non-technical language, information should be tailored to the needs of the individual and provided accordingly. The patient may need an interpreter in order to understand what is being said. The health professional must ensure interpreters are provided if required, and that appropriate written information is available to reinforce the main points.

'One stop' local anaesthesia minor operations clinic

First Appointment - Any Hospital

Dear

An appointment has been made for you to attend the ODU (Operating Day Unit) Department to see .... or a member of the team on Monday .... 2007 at 13:30.

Please bring this letter with you and report to Ward D0, which is located on the ground floor, halfway down the main corridor.

This is a one-stop clinic, which means you will be seen by the Consultant, or a specialist nurse and if you are suitable, the operation will be performed there and then under local anaesthesia.

If you are unable to attend please telephone ----------- (Mon - Fri 8am - 6pm) to arrange an alternative appointment.

Any Hospital is a teaching hospital for medical students. If you do not wish to be examined additionally by a medical student, please let us know in the clinic.

Please note that there is a Pay on Foot car park in operation. Current charges are £2 for 6 hours and £10 for 6 to 24 hours. There will be a free 20 minute drop off/pick-up time on all visitor's car parks. Disabled Badge holders can park free of charge.

Any Hospital operates a 'No Smoking' policy.

Yours sincerely

Figure 8.1 Preliminary information for the patient.

Having a Minor Operative procedure

The local anaesthetic injection may cause you slight discomfort depending on where it is given, but this discomfort lasts only a few moments.

You may still be aware of touching and pulling sensations during the procedure as the anaesthetic numbness removes only pain. The numbness will last approximately 45–60 minutes.

Any surgery to the skin will lead to some form of scar. Some scars particularly on the shoulders and upper back and chest may become sore, red and itchy temporarily, and can be treated. Other scars can spread and become wider over time. However, we are not able to do anything to prevent this.

You may experience some numbness, altered sensations or pins and needles near or around the wound after surgery. This is because small nerves in the skin are inevitably cut during surgery. These symptoms can persist for weeks or even months.

If you are taking Warfarin or Aspirin this may increase the risk of bleeding during and after your operation.

Wound infections are uncommon, but if they do occur must be treated as soon as possible with an oral antibiotic to prevent serious damage and a subsequent poor cosmetic result. Persistent pain and redness may be an indication of a wound infection.

A reaction to the materials used in the sutures (stitches) is unusual. Reactions are unpredictable and can occur many weeks after surgery. They are more likely to occur with long-lasting suture materials that are left in the skin for support purposes. A reaction may manifest itself as a persistent or growing lump.

Figure 8.2 Having a minor operative procedure. *Source*: Reproduced by kind permission of the Department of Dermatology, Royal Berkshire Hospital.

NON-VERBAL COMMUNICATION

This forms an integral part of good communication. During the initial interview, the health professional will be required to observe for non-verbal messages such as body language and eye movements. These will provide valuable clues as to how the patient is feeling, whether they are anxious or not about the impending surgery or have any other concerns.

VERBAL COMMUNICATION

It is important to speak clearly without the use of medical jargon, and to use active listening skills. Attentive listening should be followed by open-ended questions to gather more useful information, giving the patient the opportunity to ask questions (Brearley 1990). Also, by carefully listening to the patient the health professional can assess and pitch any following communication at the level that can be more readily understood. It is important to ensure that the patient fully understands by asking if they do, by pausing frequently and repeating the most salient points if necessary.

For a more detailed discussion of communication please see chapter 6.

CONSENT

'Consent is the voluntary and continuing permission of the patient to receive a particular treatment based on adequate knowledge of the purpose, nature and likely risks of the treatment including the likelihood of its success and any alternatives to it. Permission given under any unfair or undue pressure is not consent.'

(Department of Health 2003)

Types of consent can be categorised as implied or express, verbal, or written.

IMPLIED OR EXPRESS CONSENT

Consent may be expressly given in writing or orally. Alternatively, a patient through their actions may signify consent. A patient offering their wrist to have a cannula inserted, for example, is a good indication that they are giving consent to have it done.

VERBAL CONSENT

Here the patient clearly and explicitly says they agree with the proposed treatment. It is important that the patient is given the opportunity to ask questions and that the potential risks and benefits are discussed. With this type of consent, it may be advisable to document the discussion.

WRITTEN CONSENT

Here the patient's signature provides documentary evidence that they agree with the proposed procedure or treatment. However, the signature alone is not considered to be proof of consent and the patient's approval may need to be reaffirmed immediately prior to the procedure. Documentation of the consent process in the patient's notes is strongly advised.

The range of guidance documents on consent developed for use by health professionals should be consulted for details of the law and to support good practice. Failure to obtain informed consent is taken very seriously by professional regulatory bodies since, in law, any examination, treatment or investigation carried out without consent may amount to assault, which could result in an action for damages or even criminal proceedings. It is good practice to get signed consent, particularly when an intervention such as surgery is to be carried out. Consent implies that there is some choice, without which it is not valid. Validity also depends on the quality of information given.

The Kennedy Report (2001) made several recommendations on consent. Information should be tailored to the needs, circumstances and wishes of the individual, suggesting also that patients should be involved wherever possible in decisions about their treatment. The House of Lords decision in *Chester* v. *Afshar*, referred to earlier has also emphasised that extreme care must be taken in obtaining consent, and careful and comprehensive warnings about significant possible adverse outcomes must be given. These warnings must be properly recorded in the notes and the patient should be invited to sign the relevant entry to confirm that they have been given the warning, have understood it and accepts the risk.

It is equally important to make a full entry in the notes, preferably signed by the patient, if treatment is refused including the reason, if possible (NHSLA 2004).

THE LEGAL FRAMEWORK

Consent is a significant issue in the number of claims for clinical negligence, so it is important for non-medically trained healthcare personnel to 'get it right'. Where a nurse performs a role previously undertaken by a medical practitioner, the competence required to perform that role is that of the level of the medical practitioner.

The purpose of consent is to enlist the patient's faith and confidence in the efficacy of the treatment and also to provide a legal framework to protect those treating patients from a claim of damages for trespass to the person or a criminal charge of assault. However, obtaining consent does not provide a defence for negligence in either advice given or the manner in which the procedure has been carried out.

The health professional carrying out the procedure is ultimately responsible for ensuring that the patient is genuinely consenting to what is being done. It is they who will be held responsible in law if the validity of the consent is challenged later. It is a requirement that the healthcare professional providing the information must be competent to do so, especially if it is they who are carrying out the procedure. Guidance is available from professional bodies regarding consent and it is strongly suggested each practitioner discusses the area of consent with their employers to ensure they are covered by vicarious liability and that the appropriate terms and conditions are in their contract of employment, since any employee who failed to follow the legal principles relating to consent could face criminal, civil, professional conduct and disciplinary proceedings.

TRAINING ISSUES

The general system for obtaining consent should be sound and based on policy supported by staff training programmes (Pennels 2001). All trusts should have had the model consent policy in place since 1 October 2002. The Clinical Negligence Schemes for Trusts (CNST) assessments are focused on ensuring that the consent process, whether delegated or not, is audited for compliance with the model policy. If a trust decides that the consent process is not to be delegated, this should be clearly stated within the policy. Where the consent process has been delegated to staff other than the health professional capable of performing the procedure this must be clearly stated in the policy. This has several implications for the nurse obtaining consent for minor surgery.

Each Trust will have to demonstrate the following.

- Appropriate training has been undertaken.
- Practitioners are competent to perform the delegated duty and are assessed.
- An audit of the consent process (this should include appropriate documentation of discussion with the patient).
- The maintenance of a register showing which staff can perform what procedures and dates to which they apply.
- A record of who has received the appropriate training.

Each professional should ensure they are familiar with the risk assessment policies of their department and the consent training process. This should include the development of a consent training package indicating that the professional has had the appropriate training to take consent and carry out minor surgical procedures competently. It is legally possible for other healthcare professionals to obtain consent for procedures being carried out by doctors and this should be regarded as expanded role activity (Dimond 2003). It therefore follows that the person giving the information to the patient must fully understand what is proposed and must have the ability to explain to the patient, in words which they can understand, the nature of the proposed operation, the associated risks, and the alternatives, and be able to answer any questions the patient may have. Great care is necessary to ensure the patient is not given any inaccurate information or false assurances.

A delegated consent proforma should exist for the taking of consent for procedures which the professional is not trained to carry out, and this should be completed in conjunction with the Consultant Surgeon. This record, along with the training process, should be available so that the risk management department has a record or a copy of this for CNST and legal purposes. (Examples of the documentation referred to above are given in Apendices 8.1–8.5.)

GOOD PRACTICE IN CONSENT

With the introduction of the National Health Service Plan (DH 2000) patients are now being encouraged to make real choices about their care and treatment. The Department of Health has produced four model consent forms available in a variety of languages. These forms are part of the Good Practice in Consent initiative and should have been adopted by all NHS Trusts since October 2002.

These consent forms are specifically designed to meet the needs of different groups of patients, and practitioners should familiarise themselves with them. The forms now allow for the involvement of relatives and carers when making healthcare decisions and for this involvement to be documented. Where the consequences of having or not having the treatment are potentially dangerous or there is a concern for incapacitated adults, a court declaration may be sought in the patient's best interests. The four new consent forms are summarised below.

Consent Form 1 is for patients who are able to consent for themselves or who have the capacity to consent to some interventions but not to others. The procedure will involve the patient having a general anaesthetic, local anaesthetic or a sedative.

Consent Form 2 is for those with parental responsibility who are consenting on behalf of a child or young person. Those with parental responsibility include:

- the child's parents if they were married to each other at the time of conception or birth;
- the child's mother if the parents were not married at the time of conception or birth, but not necessarily the father;
- a legally appointed guardian;

- a local authority or other authorised person who has a care order or emergency protection order (MPS 2003, p 6).

Consent Form 3 is for patients who are able to consent for themselves and also for those with parental responsibility consenting on behalf of a child or young person. These are for procedures where the patients' consciousness is not impaired. Hence, this form is shorter than the others not requiring the depth of information covered in Forms 1 and 2. Therefore these are generally the most suitable for use when carrying out minor surgical procedures under local anaesthesia.

Consent Form 4 is for adults who are unable to consent to investigation or treatment. These patients are said to lack the capacity to consent and may only be treated if that treatment is believed to be in their 'best interests'. This form should ideally be completed by two doctors, and by those who are close to the patient such as relatives, spouse, carers, etc. The form contains a section for the assessment of the patient's capacity, requiring health professionals to document how judgments are reached, which colleagues have been consulted and why the procedure is considered to be in the patient's best interests.

CHILDREN AND YOUNG PEOPLE

Children may be unable to give consent for several reasons. These include difficulty in understanding the effects of their condition or the planned treatment. In most cases, persons with parental responsibility may give consent. In some circumstances consent may be given by a court. People with parental responsibility can also delegate some aspects of care to others such as childminders or boarding school staff (MPS 2003). It is advised, however, that if the health professional is in any doubt about who has parental responsibility, they should make specific enquiries.

THE GILLICK COMPETENT CHILD

This refers to a child of any age who has sufficient intelligence to fully understand the proposed treatment and could therefore give valid consent to treatment without the involvement of parents. The term *Gillick Competent* refers to the case of a woman who sought an assurance from the local health authority that her daughters would not receive advice or prescriptions without her consent. When this was refused, she challenged the legality of the decision in a case that went to the House of Lords for a final ruling. Two major principles emerged known as the Fraser Guidelines, which establish that a parent's right to consent to treatment on behalf of a child ends when the child has enough intelligence and understanding to consent for themselves and that it is for the doctor to decide whether a child has reached that level (MPS 2003). This ruling has important implications since the health professional must be clear that the child's level of understanding relates to the nature of the decision to be made (Dimond 2003).

It is assumed, unless there are good reasons to believe otherwise, that adult patients are competent to make decisions about their own affairs, including whether to give or withold their consent to medical treatment.

Patients who have difficulty retaining information or who demonstrate fluctuating competence should be given all the assistance they need to reach an informed decision.

INABILITY TO GIVE CONSENT

Many situations can arise during which a patient's ability to make healthcare decisions may be called into question, rightly or wrongly. These include:

- the premedicated patient;
- the patient in labour;
- the patient under stress;
- the patient with a known mental illness;
- the patient with organic brain disease;
- the immature patient, for example, a child or one having immature mental capacity such as some forms of mental handicap.

REFUSAL OF CONSENT

An important principle in the consent process includes the right of the patient to change their mind. The NMC (2004) maintains that any refusal of treatment or care must be respected provided it is given when the patient is legally competent. Patients can withdraw their consent at any time, but they need to be competent in order to do this. The Medical Protection Society's advice is that a patient's cry of pain during a procedure is not necessarily a withdrawal of consent and your reassurance may be enough to allow you to continue. However, if patients do object, if possible you should stop the procedure, find out their concerns and explain the consequences of not proceeding.

INFORMED CONSENT IN MINOR SURGERY

Patients have a fundamental legal and ethical right to determine what happens to their body, and therefore valid consent to treatment is absolutely necessary in all forms of healthcare (DH 2001). It is the duty of the health professional to inform the patient about any treatment and to obtain the patient's consent either verbally or in writing prior to undertaking any procedure.

Consent is a patient's agreement for a health professional to provide care and in order to be valid, the patient must:

- be competent to make the decision;
- have received enough information to make it;
- not be acting under duress.

It is very important to make sure the patient understands the procedure you intend to carry out and the possible outcomes. It is also essential that the patient is fully aware of the nature of your non-medical background. Communicating to patients and other healthcare professionals what the role involves is also essential (Younger 2006). In providing advice Younger (2006) suggests that during the initial meeting with the patient surgical care practitioners should ensure transparency and say that they are not a doctor but an SCP. The initial discussion should include a description of the intended procedure, the risks, benefits and any postoperative complications, especially any cosmetic effects.

Stem (1997) suggests the following components are required to provide the patient with pertinent information to make an intelligent, informed decision, including:

- the full diagnosis;
- a description of the proposed treatment or procedure;
- names and qualifications of those performing the procedure;
- a discussion of the potential risks and benefits;
- information on the probability of the success of the procedure;
- an explanation of discomfort or dangerous side effects the patient may experience during or after the procedure;
- an explanation of alternative methods of treatment;
- possible consequences of not having the procedure;
- awareness of the right to refuse treatment;
- awareness of the right to change their mind even after consent has been given.

The decision to operate should be reached with the patient after assessment (for example) of the site and nature of the lesion. This can then be documented in the consent form and by writing legibly in the patient's notes. The presence of the consent form in the notes supported by good documentation of the process is some proof that the healthcare professional engaged the patient in discussion about the proposed treatment.

FILLING IN THE CONSENT FORM

The consent form itself should be completed by the health professional in clear legible writing and in words that the patient can understand. There should be no abbreviations, since these can confer different meanings and cause confusion. The completed form should be read carefully by the patient and agreed by them before signing. The health professional should also sign and date the form before giving the patient a copy. The form is then stored in the patient records.

WRITTEN INFORMATION

It is usually appropriate for the patient to be given written information about the proposed procedure including the preoperative phase. Traditionally, minor operations are seen to be reasonably 'safe' procedures, which do not require as much input in terms of information and preoperative assessment as do more intermediate or major surgical procedures. However, a minor procedure may not be seen as being 'minor' to a patient who is anxious and nervous about the whole experience. It is therefore essential the health professional adopts a sympathetic and unhurried approach, taking time to explain things more than once if necessary. This provides the basis for obtaining informed consent.

Written information should also accompany any verbal discussion that takes place and this should be documented in the patient's notes. The importance of keeping up to date, legible and accurate written information should not be underestimated, particularly with the development of these new extended roles. If specific patient information on minor surgical procedures is available, this should be given at appropriate stages throughout the patient journey. If these items are not available, written information will need to be developed using the appropriate tools and networking with colleagues and peers.

FOLLOW-UP CARE

Please remember that when carrying out minor operations such as 'lumps and bumps', things can still go terribly wrong. Any invasive procedure can result in serious complications. The patient is of paramount importance, so if you are at all unsure about something ask for advice before doing it. If you make a mistake it is vital to get help and advice before you send the patient home.

If you are worried, then arrange to see the patient again within the next few days, taking time to record the patient's telephone number and phone them the following day if necessary. Follow-up is very important and can mean the difference between poor quality and excellent postoperative care.

Always ensure the patient has written information to take home following the procedure. This should include a copy of the consent form, which has documented evidence of what they actually had done, and a copy of the appropriate going home form to forward to their GP, and any postoperative instructions or information sheets (see Figures 8.3 and 8.4).

The patient may need a follow-up visit by another healthcare professional, for example, a district nurse who may need to change dressings or remove packs and drains. Specific instructions need to be accurately documented

Bleeding
Altered sensation
Impaired healing
Scarring
Infection
Keloid scar formation
Recurrence
Pain

The final cosmetic result cannot be guaranteed since every patient has a completely different healing process as far as final scar appearance is concerned

Figure 8.3 Complications of minor surgery.

and passed on to the relevant agency to ensure continuity of care. The patient should also be provided with contact details and where to attend in the case of an emergency.

TELEPHONE FOLLOW-UP

Follow-up of patients post procedure is good practice, providing continuity of care, quality and measurable outcomes, which can then be used for audit purposes. By offering a follow-up outpatient appointment the healthcare professional can provide valuable care to patients who may require further treatment. However, this may not always be possible and many patients are discharged after the initial treatment is carried out. Postoperative complications, if they do occur, are normally seen in the GP's surgery or in the A & E department, particularly if they present as an acute episode. Often there is no system to record the incidence of postoperative complications and to gather information on the patient's general experience of the service.

One way to ensure that all patients are followed up consistently is by carrying out postoperative telephone follow-up. Patients appreciate being followed up, and questions relating to the procedure and postoperative outcome will often yield very interesting information about the service itself and provide valuable feedback for audit purposes, service redesign and service improvement.

CONCLUSIONS

As nurses continue to push the boundaries in developing their roles to become autonomous practitioners, it is in their interest to 'get it right', making sure they are legally covered. Valid consent to treatment involves a patient's agreement to the intervention following a discussion and understanding of the risks and benefits of the procedure being carried out. It is absolutely vital that nurses or other healthcare professionals undertaking any extension to their

Operating Day Unit

Name:
Unit Number:
Date:
Minor Operation/Procedure Performed:

At Home:
Try to take it easy for the remainder of the day.
If possible keep the affected part elevated. For example, rest arm/leg on pillow.
You may bath or shower after 24 hours. Do not use scented salts, oils or talcum powder.
Keep the operative site as dry as possible.

Pain:
The local anaesthetic will wear off in a couple of hours.
You should be able to control any discomfort or aching by taking the tablets you would normally take for a headache, for example, paracetamol.
If you feel excessive pain please contact you family doctor.

Stitches:
Please go to your family doctor or the practice nurse to have your stiches removed in ----- days.

Follow-Up:
Normally we do not need to see you again and will refer you back to the care of your family doctor. They will be informed of the results of any histology, tests or investigations. The healthcare professional may telephone you in the next two to three weeks to see how you are getting on and answer any questions you may have regarding the procedure.

Return to Work:
Following most minor surgery we do not normally expect that you will need time off work. However this depends on what procedure you have had done and the nature of your work. If you need a sick note, please see your family doctor.

If you have concerns or worries you may contact a member of staff on the unit here on-(phone number)---
On any weekday between 08.30 am-4.30 pm
If you feel it is urgent then please return to the Accident and Emergency Department at any time during the day or night, if not you can always go to your family doctor.

Figure 8.4 Postoperative advice to the patient.

role ensure they are competent (having received the appropriate training) and that they are covered by their employing Trust to do so.

Patients require a variety of written and verbal information, and it is necessary to ensure this is available, and if not to develop systems for delivery, making use of all the available guidelines that exist and by networking so you do not have to reinvent the wheel.

If unsure about any aspect of the work you are doing, seek advice or refer your patient for more senior advice or treatment.

 Pay particular attention to how you communicate, making sure you give the patient time to absorb information and to ask questions.

Appendix 8.1

Flow chart for delegation of consent

The Consultant's agreement and involvement
□
Specify which procedures/treatments will be delegated
□
Agree criteria for measuring level of competency and monitoring of Health Care Professional
□
Agree criteria of Patients suitable for delegated consent process
□
Agree/Develop patient information leaflet and audit proforma
□
Develop training programme, gain approval from the Consent Committee's training sub group
□
Deliver training, assess competency and approve health care professional for identified agreed procedures/treatments
□
Evaluate professional and procedure by agreed processes

Appendix 8.2

Delegated consent approval record

Name of person taking delegated consent	
Procedure	
Consultant carrying out procedure	
Consultant method of carrying out procedure	
Risks	
Side effects	
Benefits	
Treatment options	
Date practitioner approved to take delegated consent	

Date for Review of Competency	
Signature of Consultant who will be carrying out procedures/ treatments	
Signature of Health Care Practitioner taking delegated Consent	

Appendix 8.3

Trust register of health care professionals who are competent to take delegated consent

Name	Division/Area	Approval Date	Review Date

Register to be maintained by Senior manager and updates forwarded to Professional Head

Appendix 8.4

Informed consent checklist

Patient information	Operation/procedure/treatment

1. Does the patient know what procedure/operation they are having? YES/NO Comments
2. Do the patient understand what will happen? YES/NO Please record patients own words of what will occur
3. Is the patient able to discuss the risks/complications as explained YES/NO Please record patients own words of the possible risks that may occur during or following treatment
4. Does the patient need to have more information about the procedure/ treatment to fully understand the risks, benefits or alternatives to treatment proposed? YES/NO Please record patients own words of what they understand to be the risks, benefits or alternative treatments
5. Does the patient require additional information to make an informed decision to consent to the procedure? YES/NO Please record patients own words of what further information they would like
6. Is the patient happy to sign the consent form YES/NO Comments
Patient signature (agreeing their comments/understanding)............
Signature of Health Care Professional taking delegated consent..... .... Date...

Appendix 8.5

Department/division delegated procedures list

Procedure/ Investigation	Department	Name of Person taking Consent	Training programme in place (Yes/No)	Staff trained (as per GMC/Trust requirement)

ACKNOWLEDGEMENTS

Appendix 8.1–8.5, reproduced by kind permission of Sandwell & West Birmingham Hospitals. Incident/Hazard Reporting Policy.

REFERENCES

Brearley S (1990) *Patient Participation: The Literature*. Harrow: Scutari Press.
Department of Health (2000) *The NHS Plan: A Plan for Investment, A Plan for Reform*. London: DH.
Department of Health (2001) *Good Practice in Consent Implementation Guide: Consent to Examination or Treatment*. London: DH.

Department of Health (2003) *Toolkit for Producing Patient Information*. London: DH.

Dimond B (2003) *Legal Aspects of Consent*. British Journal of Nursing Monograph. Wiltshire: Quay Books Division.

Gledhill L (2005) In Oxtoby (K) (2005) Consent: Obtaining Permission to Care *Nursing Times* Jan 2005, Vol 101, No 1.

Kennedy I (2001) *Bristol Royal Infirmary Inquiry. Learning from Bristol*. Report of the public inquiry into children's heart surgery at the Bristol Royal Infirmary 1984–1995. Command Paper CM 5207. London: Stationery Office.

Medical Protection Society (2003) *Consent: A Complete Guide for Students*. London: MPS.

National Health Service Litigation Authority (2004) *The CNST General Clinical Risk Management Standards* Issue 4. London: NHSLA.

Nursing and Midwifery Council (2004) *Code of Professional Conduct*. London: NMC.

Oxtoby K (2005) Consent: obtaining permission to care. *Nursing Times* **101** (1), 22–24.

Pennels C (2001) Obtaining consent: the use of a consent form. *Professional Nurse* **16** (10), 1433–1434.

Stem J (1997) Informed consent: concepts and elements. http://www.jackstem.com/informed-consent.htm(accessed 21/9/05).

Sutherland E (1996) *Day Surgery: A Handbook for Nurses*. London: Bailliere Tindall.

Tingle J (1998) Legal aspects of expanded roles and clinical guidelines and protocols. In: McHale J, Tingle J, and Peysner J, *Law and Nursing*. Oxford: Butterworth Heinemann.

United Kingdom Central Council (1992) *The Scope of Professional Practice*. London: UKCC.

Younger J (2006) More on the surgical care practitioner role. *The Clinical Services Journal*.

ESSENTIAL READING

Department of Health (2003) *12 Key Points on Consent: the Law in England*. London: DH.

Dimond B (2001) *Legal Aspects of Nursing* (3rd edn). London: Pearson Education.

Tingle J (1998) Legal aspects of expanded role and clinical guidelines and protocols. In: McHale J, Tingle J and Peysner J (1998) *Law and Nursing*. Oxford: Butterworth Heinemann.

National Association of Assistants in Surgical Practice (2005) *The NAASP Law & Consent Course for Healthcare Professionals: Course Handbook*. London: NAASP.

USEFUL WEBSITE ADDRESSES

Department of Health
Policy documents
http://www.doh.gov.uk

National Association of Assistants in Surgical Practice
www.NAASP.org.uk

Nursing and Midwifery Council
Regulatory, professional and educational information
www.nmc-uk.og.uk

Royal College of Nursing
Employment and professional issues
www.rcn.org.uk

9 Documentation

ANURAG PATEL AND SANJAY PURKAYASTHA

Documentation is a vital part of medical practice, being one of many facets of clinical governance. Regular review and audit should be undertaken to raise standards, which are frequently lower than the ideal.

It is important to appreciate that documentation, although important in a medico-legal setting, should not be carried out only for this purpose. It is a prime communication tool for your patient's care, and efforts should be made to optimise the quality of note-keeping in all medical settings. As an example, Bateman et al. (*J R Coll Surg Edinb* 1999, 44(2), 94–5) greatly improved the standards of documentation in surgical operative notes within their Otolaryngology/Head and Neck Unit by providing an aide memoire, simply attaching this to the operation note. The result was a significant decrease in the use of unacceptable abbreviations and difficulties in identifying the operating surgeon.

Ploughing through many pages in a patient's notes is very tedious but it is necessary in carrying out audit and research. Development of paper-free medical records is the future. Electronic methods will enable quick and easy access on a daily basis to such areas as date on patient records, investigation results or radiological images, thus adding to the improvement of patient care.

Providing mobile data retrieval facilities will introduce a new era in electronic access to patient records. It is intended to install such facilities in all cardiology departments in the United States in accordance with the recommendation of the American College of Cardiology. A study in 2002 by Burkle et al. (*Stud Health Technol Inform* 2002; 90, 256–61) within their Endoscopy Department found that although guideline-based documentation may not be suitable for all endoscopy cases, such documentation that is properly structured can generate essential classification codes. This can improve the harvesting of information for conducting research. However, a question remains as to whether an electronic based system can provide an option to input patient data in narrative format. Certain patients will fit the criteria for inputting information in a proforma format enabling the production of an automatic narrative report but it is important that facilities are in place to prevent the loss of valuable patient information, as not all patients will fit the 'box'.

Minor Surgical Procedures for Nurses and Allied Healthcare Professionals. Edited by Shirley Martin.
© 2007 John Wiley & Sons Limited

Consistency and thoroughness of documentation remains substandard and standards must be improved and audited regularly. Following established guidelines can help this. Patel et al.'s audit of documentation in hospital medical notes within surgical units in two hospitals found that on average only two thirds of the entries specified by The Royal College of Surgeons of England guidelines were present and correct (*Ann R Coll Surg Engl* 1993; 75 (1), 7–9). Substandard categories included regular update of notes, postoperative instructions, comments about postoperative recovery, the record of advice given to relatives, and incorrect consent.

There is an array of guidelines available, of which a few are mentioned in this chapter. It is important when developing integrated care pathways (ICPs) to incorporate this guidance to ensure satisfactory documentation. In an audit comparing traditional note-keeping and ICPs in an orthopaedic unit, Crawford and Shanahan (*Ann R Coll Surg Engl* 2003; 85(3), 197–9) found that although both groups had high frequency of omissions, the quality of record keeping was higher when using the traditional notation system.

Maintaining standards of note-keeping should be checked out by audit. A useful system is the CRABEL score developed by Crawford, Beresford and Lafferty which was introduced in 2001 for auditing medical note-keeping at Morriston Hospital, Swansea. In 2004 Dhariwal and Gibbons published work using this system (*Br J Oral Maxillofac Surg* 2004; 42(3):200–2). They found that the CRABEL score was simple, reliable and repeatable when auditing note-keeping in their maxillofacial unit. They felt it a successful and objective measure for audit and for improvement in the quality of note-keeping.

The General Medical Council's 'good medical practice' guidelines state that medical records should be 'clear, accurate, legible and contemporaneous'. They further state that one should report 'relevant clinical findings, decisions made, information given to the patient, and any drugs or treatment provided'.

The Royal College of Surgeons of England has provided the following 'guidelines for clinicians on medical records and notes':

1 The hospital record

Up to date identification data must be maintained for every patient:

1. A unique medical record number or reference on every page.
2. Name in full on every page.
3. Address and post code.
4. Telephone number.
5. Date of birth.
6. Sex.
7. Next of kin details.
8. Occupation and marital status.
9. The patient's registered general practitioner.

2 Clinical record keeping

Notes should contain:
1. an initial patient history with details of previous illnesses, the social and environmental context of the illness when appropriate, and details of medication;
2. details of the initial physical examination, including the patient's height and weight;
3. a working diagnosis and medical care plan.

Notes should be supplemented and updated regularly to include details and reports of all investigations, treatments and verbal advice given to the patient and/or their relatives.

An entry must be made on discharge recording the clinician responsible for the decision to discharge, the status and destination of the patient and arrangements for follow-up. A copy of the preliminary discharge letter should be filed in the notes.

3 Patients undergoing surgery

Records should include the following details.
1. Signed evidence that informed consent has been obtained by a doctor or an appropriately trained nurse practitioner.
2. Signed evidence that the correct procedure was followed when obtaining consent for children under the age of 16 years.
3. The medical care plan, including the site and side of any operative procedure. Sites and sides must be written out in full and not abbreviated.

An operative record made immediately postoperatively should include the information listed below.
1. Name of the operating surgeon(s) and the name of the consultant responsible.
2. Diagnosis made and the procedure performed.
3. Description of the findings.
4. Details of tissues removed, altered or added.
5. Details of serial numbers of prosthetics used.
6. Details of sutures used.
7. An accurate description of any difficulties or complications encountered and how these were overcome.
8. Immediate postoperative instructions.
9. Surgeon's signature.

4 Details on discharge

The Medical Defence Union has also provided advice on good record keeping which provides a useful adjunct to the RCSE's guidelines. The advice is based on the guidelines set out by the General Medical Council's Good Medical Practice booklet, summarised below.

- Avoid abbreviations. If you do use them, use only approved unambiguous abbreviations. Left and right should always be written in full.
- Avoid personal comments. A flippant remark in the notes may make it difficult to convince a judge of a professional clinical approach.
- Give adequate details on request forms for pathology, X-rays, etc. Ensure they are signed and dated.
- See, evaluate and initial reports before they are filed in the patient's records. Make a note of abnormal results and record any action.
- Check dictated notes and sign them.
- Write legibly and print your name.
- Do not erase, overwrite or tippex out notes. They should be scored out with a single line and the corrected entry written alongside with a date, time and signature. Any additions should be separately dated, timed and signed. Never try to insert new notes.
- Always note the date and time of an entry. This may be vital medico-legally in the event of a claim.

Many lessons can be learnt from medico-legal cases and it is imperative that suggestions for improvements are incorporated into everyday practice. Further areas where documentation must be improved include:

- when the patient is unknown to the doctor detailed factual information about the patient must be recorded at the point of contact;
- verification of the information at appropriate intervals;
- when documenting it is important that the practitioner records all their relevant concerns without venturing into speculation that cannot be justified;
- records of discussions must include relevant telephone conversations, any departmental meetings in which the patient is discussed (eg multidisciplinary meetings);
- when a practitioner is working in situations where the case notes are not available any relevant information should be entered in the notes as soon as practicable.

For further information and a good example of a Trust-based guideline please refer to http://www.addenbrookes.org.uk/advice/medethlaw.

REFERENCES

Bateman ND, Carney AS, Gibbin KP (1999) 'An audit of the quality of operation notes in an otolaryngology unit.' *J R Coll Surg Edinburgh*. Apr; **44**(2), 94–5.
Burkle T, Ganslandt T, Tubergen D, Mengel J, Kuchargik T, et al (2002) 'Guideline based structured documentation: the final goal?' *Stud Health Technol Inform*. **90**, 256–61.

Part Three
Clinical Practices

10 Maintaining Asepsis: Preventing Infection of the Surgical Site

CHRISTINE MCDOUGALL

The purpose of asepsis is to prevent bacterial contamination of the open surgical wound by isolating it within a sterile field in a controlled surgical environment. It should be the primary aim of everyone working in any surgical location in both hospital and primary care setting.

It is difficult to define 'minor surgery' because an increasing range of surgical procedures are performed by practitioners who are not surgeons, and many of these are carried out in facilities that are not purpose-built operating theatres. Whilst there are evidence based guidelines for prevention of surgical site infection (Mangram et al. 1999; Woodhead et al. 2002) there is limited research or published information on infection rates for minor surgery. Therefore best practice should be based on closely related guidance and risk assessment.

Surgical wound infections resulting in sepsis and death were common before Joseph Lister introduced the concept of antisepsis in 1867, and despite continuing advances in both aseptic practices and surgical environments, they remain one of the most common healthcare associated infections. This could be explained by the increasing complexity of surgery and use of implants, and the numbers of patients undergoing surgery who are at increased risk of infection due to underlying conditions. Sepsis and death are less common but these infections continue to have a serious impact on patients and the health service and although this impact varies depending on the type of surgery (Coello et al. 2005) it remains an undesirable and expensive outcome (Plowman et al. 2001).

Mangram et al. (1999) suggest that many of these infections can be prevented by identifying the risks that increase the likelihood of infection and managing them in a realistic way. Woodhead et al. (2002) have identified four important factors that determine wound infection: the degree of bacterial contamination of the wound, the virulence of the bacteria, the amount of tissue trauma, and the immune response of the patient. Therefore prevention depends on both surgical skill and an understanding of the physical and

Minor Surgical Procedures for Nurses and Allied Healthcare Professionals. Edited by Shirley Martin.
© 2007 John Wiley & Sons Limited

environmental measures that are important in preventing bacterial contamination of the wound.

This chapter will cover these issues under the following headings:

Recognising the risks

Intrinsic and extrinsic risk factors.
Bacterial sources.

Managing the risks

1. Managing the patient at risk.
2. Environmental controls.
   Ventilation.
   Theatre attire.
   Building design and environmental issues.
   Cleaning.
3. Decontamination of surgical instruments.
   Disposable instruments.
   Contracting out.
   Reprocessing reusable instruments.
4. Maintaining asepsis in the sterile field.
   Surgical scrub.
   Gloving and gowning.
   Laying up and maintaining a sterile field.
   Skin prep and drapes.

RECOGNISING THE RISKS

EXTRINSIC AND INTRINSIC RISK FACTORS

The likelihood of surgical site infection is influenced by intrinsic and extrinsic risk factors (Garibaldi et al. 1991).

Intrinsic factors are those related to the patient that can affect healing and the ability to resist infection, for example, age, diabetes, heart disease, immune suppression, obesity or malnutrition. As much as possible, attempts should be made to target measures to reduce some of these risks preoperatively.

There are two major extrinsic factors, environmental and procedural. Environmental risks are associated with the risk of exogenous bacterial contamination of the wound (see Bacterial sources) and are affected by premises and ventilation, equipment, the surgical team and theatre protocols.

Procedural risks are associated with the surgical technique in maintaining asepsis and minimising tissue damage. Leaper (1995) suggests that surgeons who are gentle reduce the risk of infection because they minimise tissue trauma, cause less bleeding and formation of haematoma and prevent dead space and desiccation of tissue.

BACTERIAL SOURCES

Bacteria that cause surgical wound infection come from two major sources: the patient's own bacterial flora (endogenous) and sources such as theatre staff, equipment or the operating environment (exogenous).

Endogenous contamination originates from the patient's skin, nose, and other parts of the body that are naturally colonised with bacteria; the gastro-intestinal tract, genitourinary tract and upper respiratory tract. These 'normal body flora' do no harm in their normal location. However, they may invade the tissues during a surgical procedure. The risk depends on the anatomical site of the operation and can be predicted by the 'wound class' (Mangram et al. 1999) which distinguishes clean, clean contaminated, contaminated, and dirty wounds, based on the degree of microbial contamination likely to be present in the wound at the time of surgery. Most minor surgical procedures will be classed as 'clean', defined as procedures in which there is no inflam-mation or open trauma and the operation does not involve entry into the respiratory, alimentary, or genitourinary tract, with primary wound closure and closed drainage. The organisms that commonly cause infection in this class are those that originate from the skin. This can be the skin of the patient (endogenous) or the skin of the theatre staff (exogenous).

The major exogenous source is bacteria attached to skin and hair particles shed by theatre staff. These particles are airborne for a short time but can settle directly into the wound or part of the sterile field (eg instruments, gloves, drapes or gowns) and subsequently may be introduced into the wound. They can also settle as dust on horizontal surfaces, becoming airborne again when disturbed. Exogenous contamination with other microorganisms has been traced to contaminated antiseptics used for skin prep and instruments that have been inadequately decontaminated or become contaminated because principles of asepsis are not maintained.

BACTERIA OF THE SKIN

The skin forms a protective covering and is a major part of the body's defence against microbial invasion. It has three major parts: an outer layer or epider-mis, an inner layer or dermis, and appendages which are nails and hair. The epidermis is made up of layers of cells, the superficial layer of which is com-posed of dead cells, referred to as the keratin layer, which are constantly shed and replaced by the cells of the deeper layers.

The hair follicles are colonised with 'resident flora'. These are primarily made up of micrococci species, coagulase negative staphylococci,

Staphylococcus epidermidis and corynebacteria, though *Staphylococcus aureus* can colonise the skin of nasal carriers. The density and composition of skin flora vary with anatomical location, being highly concentrated in high moisture areas with hair, for example the axilla and groin, and less where the skin is dryer with less hair, for example the forearm. The area of skin around any body orifice may also be colonised with the same organisms that exist within that orifice. Therefore the perineum or groin may also be colonised with normal flora from the rectum and genitourinary tract, and skin around the mouth and nose with oral and upper respiratory tract flora.

Other microorganisms known as transient flora are acquired and transferred between the skin, environment, equipment and other people by contact. In the healthcare setting there is an increased risk that some transient flora will be resistant to commonly used antibiotics, for example methicillin resistant *Staphylococcus aureus* (MRSA).Transient flora are easily removed from the skin by washing or the use of antiseptic preparations, and from the environment by cleaning.

MANAGING THE RISKS

1.) THE PATIENT AT RISK

Any surgical patient is at risk of surgical site infection but some are more susceptible than others. Mangram et al. (1999) detail intrinsic risk factors and preventive measures, for example ensuring blood glucose control in diabetic patients, improving nutrition and hygiene and appropriate use of prophylactic antibiotics, which in minor surgery may be indicated for cases with heart disease or increased risk of infection due to immune suppression or where the wound class is other than clean.

Surgical skin preparation is described later in this chapter but it is practical to encourage patients to bathe before they attend for minor surgery. Hair that may impede the procedure should be removed, preferably with clippers immediately before skin prep. Shaving should be avoided.

Jewellery should be removed only if it is directly in the operative field. Clothing should be removed to enable sufficient exposure of the operative site and enable thorough skin prep and draping (Woodhead et al. 2002). In some cases it may be prudent to remove an item of clothing to prevent damage or staining with antiseptic. However, ensure the patient's modesty at all times.

2.) ENVIRONMENTAL CONTROLS

Environmental aspects that influence the risk of surgical site infection are operating room ventilation and design, decontamination of surgical instruments and theatre attire and protocols (Humphries, Stacey and Taylor 1995).

Ventilation

The air in any operating room may be contaminated with bacteria carrying particles or respiratory droplets from operating room staff. The level of contamination is directly proportional to the number of people present and the amount of movement that takes place (Ayliffe 1991). Other possible sources include polluted air supply, backtracking of air from adjacent rooms, disturbed dust from the environment or organisms shed from scrub suits and gowns that have become contaminated in storage or in use. The presence of specialist ventilation influences the level of contamination.

The ideal

The risk from airborne contamination is reduced in conventionally ventilated theatres by:

- filtering the supplied air to remove 90% of bacteria laden particles;
- diluting existing contamination;
- preventing the entry of polluted air from outside the operating room (Hoffman et al. 2002).

Full technical details are given in Health Technical Memorandum 2025 (NHS Estates 1994). A clearer explanation of the document has been produced for infection control teams by a working party of the Hospital Infection Society (Hoffman et al. 2002), and a paper by Chow and Yang (2004) describes how the current technical and microbiological standards for ventilated theatres have evolved.

In simple terms, a high volume of filtered air is supplied into the cleanest areas, ie the operating and preparation room, providing 15 to 20 air changes every hour and diluting contamination. This strong current of air (positive pressure) forces any airborne particles and contaminants out into less clean areas of the theatre suite, eg corridor and adjacent areas, before they can migrate to the wound or sterile field. It also prevents contaminated air flowing back into the operating room. The efficacy, however, can be affected if doors are propped open or continually being opened and closed. Practitioners working in the well designed and managed environment of the hospital operating theatre or day surgery unit should be working in the ideal operating environment. Their responsibilities are to report faults and ensure regular maintenance programmes are supported.

The acceptable

Smyth et al. (2005) suggest that although current guidelines advise on air quality and how to provide it, apart from orthopaedics it is unclear what specification of ventilation is necessary for other types of surgery. Most existing specifications, derived by expert groups, are not evidence-based because clinical trials to establish different specifications would be expensive and logistically and ethically difficult.

Two surveys of operating theatres in the UK (Humphries et al. 1995; Smyth et al. 2005) discovered that minor surgery and minimally invasive surgery are often performed in non-ventilated theatres comparable with treatment rooms. However, they advise that appropriate ventilation is only one component of a strategy to minimise infection and that for procedures other than those involving a prosthetic implant, it is less significant than other environmental factors and theatre protocols.

If a conventionally ventilated theatre is available it should be utilised, otherwise ensure the very best that can realistically be achieved. Measures listed below should be considered when using an operating room without conventional ventilation.

- Windows should be sealed closed to prevent contamination from the outside environment by bacteria carrying dust particles, insects, etc.
- Convector heaters must not be used. Solid radiators must be of a design that will not harbour and trap dust.
- Consider plume retrieval if using diathermy in a non-ventilated theatre.
- If there is any form of mechanical air supply or air cooling system in existence consult a ventilation engineer to establish the following:
  ○ that the point at which air enters the system is not at risk of contamination;
  ○ if the air is filtered, to what standard, and what maintenance contracts are in place;
  ○ if there is extraction from the room, it is not so strong that it draws air from adjacent rooms and corridors (Blowers et al. 1995).

Theatre attire

Correctly worn scrub suits and head covering control the level of bacteria laden particles shed from theatre staff (Humphries et al. 1991) and are an important element of theatre protocols outlined in relevant guidelines (Mangram et al. 1999; Woodhead et al. 2002). They are particularly important in a non-ventilated theatre in the absence of mechanical controls. Although use of face masks is controversial (Mitchell and Hunt 1991; Romney 2001), they must be worn, in addition to eye protection, for the personal protection of the operating team (Pratt et al. 2001).

If using diathermy or laser always wear correctly fitted plume masks to protect against smoke inhalation (Woodhead et al. 2002). An independent working party document also gives useful guidance and rationale for the protective properties of all theatre attire (Adams et al. 2005).

Building design and environmental issues

Research and investigation have consistently confirmed that the healthcare environment is a reservoir for microorganisms with the potential to cause infection (NHS Estates 2002). Most microorganisms can survive where dust and dirt provide nutrients, therefore the design and layout of the operating suite or minor surgery facility should be such as to minimise accumulation of dust and facilitate easy cleaning. The ideal is portrayed as a purpose built operating theatre with adjacent scrub room, laying up room, anaesthetic room, etc. Such designs are set out in guidance documents, for example NHS Estates Health Building Notes HBN 26 (2005).

For minor surgery premises outside hospital, NHS Estates provide a guidance document on planning and design in Primary and Social Care Premises (NHS Estates website). Additional recommendations are given in *Infection Control in the Built Environment* (NHS Estates 2002) which discusses the importance of 'designing in' the fundamental requirements that facilitate optimal infection control. The important issues listed below are summarised from these documents. However local infection control advice is strongly recommended.

• The operating room must be a dedicated room and not used for any other purpose, such as an office or store room.
• Surface finishes must be fluid repellent and easily cleaned with all joints and crevices sealed to prevent water egress.
• Floors, walls, furniture, all fixtures and fittings and all lighting must have smooth easy to clean surfaces.
• There must be no soft furnishings or carpet.
• No curtains, but vertical blinds that can be easily cleaned or blinds within the double glazing.
• There must be dedicated hand washing sinks or scrub sinks, with elbow operated mixer taps and sealed water proof splash backs. There should be no plug or overflow and taps must be aligned so that the water does not run directly into the drain aperture. Sinks fitted into work tops or vanity type units are not recommended. There should be no cupboards under sinks.
• Liquid soap, antiseptic scrub and paper towels must be available from wall mounted dispensers near the sink. A foot operated bin must be positioned next to the sink for disposal of paper towels.
• Separate sinks must be available for decontamination of instruments and for domestic use.
• Storage in cupboards is preferable to racking which enables dust to accumulate. Ensure there is ample storage to avoid storing surplus items inappropriately such as on the floor. Cupboards must be dry and cool and not at risk of becoming contaminated with damp or dust, or risk of damage to packaging of sterile packs.

- There must be a separate cupboard for cleaning equipment and consumables.
- Sharps bins should be attached to wall or shelf out of the reach of children.
- There should be a dedicated room designed for decontamination of surgical instruments if applicable.
- There should be safe holding areas for clinical waste, used instruments and used linen. These areas must be separate from the operating room but also be easily accessible.

Environmental cleaning

Hospital detergent and water are adequate for all routine cleaning, which should remove rather than redistribute dust and soiling. Lint free single use cloths should be used, the cleaning solution should be changed frequently and buckets, bowls and mops stored clean and dry between uses. Detergent spray with disposable cloths or detergent impregnated wipes provide a convenient alternative. Appropriate protective clothing, to include non-sterile gloves and a plastic apron, with face protection whenever there is a risk of splashing to the face, must be worn when cleaning. The following recommendations are summarised from Mangram et al. (1999) and Woodhead et al. (2002).

- All spillages and splashes of blood and body fluids must be removed as soon as possible after the procedure and the contaminated area washed with a solution of hypochlorite according to local spillage policies.
- After each case the operating table and any non-invasive items of equipment that have been used should be cleaned.
- As a routine, after the last case of the day all horizontal surfaces and equipment, including lighting, should be cleaned and the floors washed. Mop heads must be machine washed and stored dried.
- Drug cupboards and fridges should be cleaned weekly and stock rotated to ensure they are used by the given date. There should be a regular cleaning programme for all other cupboards and storage areas to prevent accumulation of dust.
- Walls should be washed every six months.

3.) DECONTAMINATION OF SURGICAL INSTRUMENTS

Inadequately decontaminated surgical instruments present a significant infection risk. It is the responsibility of the user to ensure that the equipment they intend to use is 'fit for purpose' in that it has been subjected to an appropriately validated process and that every reasonable precaution has been taken to ensure that the sterile condition of the product has been maintained up to the point of use. A working knowledge of decontamination processes is essential, even though they may be carried out by others. Practitioners working in a hospital with an 'in house Theatre Sterile Services Unit' (TSSU) must ensure local protocols for containment and transportation of used instrument packs, and storage of sterile packs are followed. Minor surgery units in the community have three options for ensuring safe instruments: using disposable instruments; contracting a sterile services provider; or reprocessing own reusable instruments. The Medical Devices Agency (2002) provides a helpful flow chart to assist in making this decision.

Whichever of these options is utilised, the following documents provide detailed advice and guidance on the many important issues that need to be addressed.

- NHS Estates (2003) A guide to the decontamination of reusable surgical instruments. This gives comprehensive information on the basic requirements for decontamination including all steps of the decontamination cycle. This information is important even if you do not intend to process your own instruments as the steps include transport and storage. It also refers to many other NHS Estates guidance documents and Medical Devices Agency documents on maintenance and testing of sonic washers, washer disinfectors, autoclaves and benchtop sterilisers.
- Medical Devices Agency (2002) *Benchtop Steam Sterilizers – Guidance on Purchase, Operation and Maintenance.*

Disposable instruments

The decision to use disposables depends on the type of surgery, availability of suitable good quality instruments and availablity of resources for decontamination of reusable instruments. Also consider the safe disposal of an increased volume of clinical waste and the costs involved. Single use instruments must never be decontaminated and re-used (Medical Devices Agency 2000).

Contracting out

Registered sterile services providers have sufficient capacity to process instruments from a number of healthcare providers and have the expertise, equipment and environment to process devices to a high standard. If this service is available, plan well to ensure a consistently adequate supply of instrument packs to your specifications in an efficient turnaround time. Consideration should also be given to safe containment, holding and transportation of used instrument packs, and delivery and storage of sterile packs.

Reprocessing reusable instruments

If the above service is not available or its use is not practicable, the same high standards must be achieved locally. This depends on a sufficient supply of instruments, good facilities for processing and influential training that expresses the importance of thorough decontamination. Practical knowledge of decontamination and the NHS Estates Guidance (2003) mentioned above is essential. There should be robust local protocols in place for every stage of the decontamination cycle. It is strongly recommended that all staff responsible for decontamination complete the NHS Estates online training course (NHS Estates 2004). Carefully consider the MDA guidance (2002) and MDA safety notice (2002 A) on purchase, operation and maintenance of sterilisers, and consult the infection control services locally to ensure suitable equipment is purchased. Ensure that validation and periodic testing of sterilisers are carried out (Medical Devices Agency 1998) and maintenance programmes are in place.

4.) MAINTAINING ASEPSIS IN THE STERILE FIELD

Asepsis is achieved by creating a sterile field in which to work, effectively isolating the surgical site from the non-sterile environment using sterile drapes gowns and gloves. It includes the draped prepared surgical site, the exposed instruments and the sterile theatre attire worn by the operator. Maintenance depends on aseptic principles that do not allow anything that is non-sterile to come into contact with any part of the sterile field (Osman 2000; Roark 2003). For minor procedures, the extent to which this is done may vary and it is the responsibility of the practitioner to make a careful assessment based on the intended surgical process, the anticipated size and depth of the surgical wound, use of implant or drain, the duration of the procedure and the susceptibility of the patient (see Table 10.1).

Stages to establish the sterile field include:

- surgical scrub and donning sterile gown and gloves, commonly known as 'scrubbed';
- laying up surgical instruments;
- skin prep and positioning surgical drapes.

Surgical scrub

Surgical hand disinfection is required to remove transient microorganisms and reduce and suppress resident flora for at least the duration of the procedure. Rings, with the exception of plain wedding rings, and wrist jewellery must be removed as these will hinder effective hand decontamination and will harbour bacteria (Hoffman et al. 2004). False nails harbour microorganisms and should not be worn in clinical practice (Hedderwick et al. 2000).

Chlorhexidine or iodine detergent preparations are available and are equally effective though the residual effect of chlorhexidine makes it a better choice. However, user acceptability should be acknowledged as skin reactions

Table 10.1 Guide to procedures and personal protective equipment

The following is intended as a guide only. The principles of aseptic technique should always be maintained, particularly the decontamination of hands, use of sterile instruments, no-touch technique and maintaining the sterile field. Personal protective equipment (PPE) should be used according to an assessment of the risk of exposure to blood and body fluids. However the use of full sterile gown and gloves; or single use plastic apron and non-sterile gloves, must be based on the risk of wound infection. Risk assessment should be based on the size and depth of the surgical incision, the likely duration of the procedure, the anticipated tissue trauma, possibility of complication, use of implant, wound drain and susceptibility of the patient to infection.

No Incision	Incision	
Removal of toe nail Cryotherapy	**Simple minor surgery** Small incision involving subcutaneous layers Short duration	**Advanced minor surgery** Larger or deeper incision required/anticipated
Injecting varicose veins	Removal of moles, skin tags	Lipoma Sebaceous cysts Ganglia Carpal tunnel Hernia Trigger Finger Circumcision
Minimal PPE	**Minimal PPE**	**Minimal PPE** Sterile gown and gloves
Clean full length plastic apron. Face protection. Sterile or clean non-sterile gloves	Clean full length plastic apron Face protection Sterile gloves	Appropriate mask Eye protection **Additional precautions** Ventilated theatre recommended for: procedures that require an incision deeper than subcutaneous layer; insertion of implant, e.g mesh

resulting in damaged skin increase the number of resident flora and the risk of transient carriage.

Surgical scrub should be carried out at a designated hand washing sink or scrub sink with elbow operated taps, and should be conducted as follows:

• surgical scrub should take place immediately before donning sterile gown and gloves;
• first scrub of the list must include thorough cleaning under the nails with a manicure stick file or brush. Scrubbing of skin with a brush is not recommended as resulting abrasions increase the risk of colonisation with transient flora;

- adjust water temperature, wet the hands, and apply the antiseptic detergent thoroughly to all aspects of the hands and forearms, continuing washing for 2–3 minutes;
- rinse hands and arms thoroughly from fingers to elbows, and then keep hands up away from the body with elbows in a flexed position so that water runs away from the tips of the fingers towards the elbows;
- dry using a sterile towel starting with the finger tips and working towards the elbows.

Alcohol hand rubs are an acceptable alternative to repeated surgical scrub after the first scrub of a list and can be used to decontaminate the hands for subsequent operative procedures. However this depends on what activities are undertaken between cases and should be assessed on the risk of hands becoming contaminated with organic matter in which case alcohol will not be effective (Hoffman et al. 2004). If used, alcohol solutions should be applied to the hands and forearms ensuring contact with all aspects of the hands until dry immediately before gowning and gloving.

All detergent and antiseptic solutions must be stored in cool, dry cupboards and used in date. Hand preparations must be available from pump dispensers. Bottles must be used until empty and never topped up or re-filled. Antiseptic solutions for preparation of the patient's skin should be supplied in single-use containers or sachets. Multi-use containers are subject to contamination once opened (Woodhead et al. 2002; Hoffman et al. 2004).

Sterile gowns, gloves and drapes

The purpose of sterile gowns and drapes is to provide a barrier that prevents transfer of microorganisms to the surgical site. They also protect the operator from exposure to patient's blood and exudates during the procedure. The efficacy depends on the fabric's ability to resist fluids. If they are not fluid repellent when they get wet with blood or other fluids bacteria can be drawn through the fabric by capillary action known as 'wicking' or 'strike through'. The European Standard for sterile theatre gowns and drapes states that these must be disposable single use items. This may be considered excessive for minor surgery where the depth of the incision and blood loss is less likely to soak the sleeves of the gown and the drapes. However each practitioner must assess their optimal requirements and select gowns and drapes accordingly. Three reports, endorsed by the Association for Perioperative Practice (AfPP), provide help in deciding on the choice of gowns and drapes (Graff et al. 2001; Garner, Graff et al. 2002; Garner, Gilmore et al. 2003).

Sterile gloves

Sterile gloves prevent transmission of microorganisms from the hands of the operating practitioner and protect the practitioner from exposure to blood and body fluids from the operative site. If gloves become damaged during a procedure they must be changed.

The technique for donning sterile gloves and gowns requires practice to establish the competency which is essential to the practitioner becoming a safe element of the sterile field. The best way to learn is to observe and seek guidance from an experienced colleague.

Laying up

The activity of arranging sterile instruments, solutions, swabs, dressings, etc., is generally called 'laying up' and normally requires two people, one scrubbed and wearing sterile gown and gloves and touching only sterile items, the other assisting by transferring and dispensing subsidiary packs and solutions on to the sterile field using methods that maintain sterility and integrity (Osman 2000). The secure surface of a trolley or table, cleaned after each case to prevent any cross infection, is essential. Instruments must be arranged on the sterile surface created from the inner layer of the instrument pack wrappings when carefully opened. Alternatively sterile drapes can be used to arrange singly wrapped sterile instruments. Laying up should be done immediately before the procedure, as exposed instruments can become contaminated with airborne particles (Humphries and Taylor 2002, Chow and Yang 2004). If there is any delay they must be covered with a sterile drape. When working alone, scrub and glove, carefully open the pack to create the sterile field, dispense solutions and subsidiary items, and cover with sterile drape. Once the patient is positioned for the proceduce decontaminate hands again and don appropriate attire.

Skin prep

The skin at the operative site should be cleaned and disinfected with an antiseptic that will remove any transient flora and reduce and repress resident flora. It should have a residual activity that lasts at least the duration of the operation, preferably longer.

Although any of the skin disinfectants in Table 10.2 can be effective the following must be considered when selecting a preoperative skin disinfectant.

- Chlorhexidine and iodine are available in aqueous or alcoholic solutions. The advantage of using an alcohol based antiseptic is that it will have a rapid effect and will dry quickly.
- Alcohol based antiseptics should be used sparingly. If used too generously and allowed to pool under the patient the alcohol may ignite when using diathermy and can cause severe burns (MDA 2000B).
- Alcohol based antiseptics are not suitable for some areas of the body as the alcohol will be irritant on the face, genital area or broken skin.

Table 10.2 Recommended preoperative skin disinfectants

Chlorhexidine	Alcohol	Iodine
Properties	**Properties**	**Properties**
Broad spectra	Broad spectra	Broad spectra
Intermediately rapid reaction	Rapid action	Intermediately rapid action
Excellent residual activity	No residual activity	Residual activity minimal
Achieves good reduction of skin flora		
Not inactivated by blood or serum protein		
Negative effect	**Negative effect**	**Negative effect**
Ototoxicity – irritant to middle ear	Drying	Can be inactivated by blood and serum proteins
Keratitis – irritant to eyes	Volatile	Absorption from skin possible with possible toxicity
	Flammable, therefore risk of burns during diathermy if it pools under patient or is not allowed to dry	Skin irritation
		Contraindicated in babies and children and during pregnancy

- Residual activity means that the antiseptic will continue to be effective for some hours after it has been applied, therefore protecting the wound from bacteria for some time after it has been closed.
- Do not use one product followed by another, eg chlorhexidine followed by iodine because they will inactivate each other.
- Always ask the patient about allergy to any of these products.

Before antiseptic skin preparation is applied the skin should be socially clean. Wash with soap and water if the patient has been unable to manage washing or there has been incontinence or other contamination with organic matter.

Apply the antiseptic with friction for 2–3 minutes in concentric circles beginning in the area of the proposed incision and working outward to include an area large enough to extend the incision should this be necessary (Hoffman et al. 2004). The skin must be allowed to dry before positioning sterile drapes.

Sterile drapes

Sterile drapes prevent transfer of microorganisms from non-sterile non-prepped skin and non-sterile adjacent areas to the intended incision site. A fenestrated drape should be used for the intended area of incision, and additional drapes placed on the patient, furniture and equipment as appropriate.

To minimise contamination of the surgical site and sterile gloves when placing drapes, the gloved hands should be protected by cuffing the drape material over the gloved hands and placing the drape from surgical site to periphery. Once in place the underside of the drape will no longer be sterile, sterility of the sterile field will be compromised if they are moved or handled (Roark 2003).

CONCLUSION

Whether minor surgery is carried out in hospital or in a community setting patients have the right to high standards of care and treatment. It is the responsibility of minor surgery practitioners to develop skilled surgical techniques and high standards of asepsis in a well maintained safe environment. Each minor surgery unit should have infection control policies that are compliant with national guidelines and best practice in association with risk assessment.

To ensure continuing standards are maintained carry out regular audits of premises and practice, ensure continuing maintenance contracts for ventilation and arrange regular inspection validation and testing of decontamination equipment. Finally monitor outcomes, particularly infection of the surgical site, and if they occur, examine practices, revisit guidelines and review policies.

REFERENCES

Adams G, Garner S, Gilmour D, et al. (2005) *Trust and Protection. Protecting Operating Theatre Staff from the Risk of Infection.* Report from an independent multidisciplinary working group. Hsdcommunications. Herts: Rickmansworth.

Ayliffe GA (1991) Role of the environment in the operating suite in surgical wound infection. *Rev. Infect. Dis.* **13** (S10): 800–804.

Blowers R, Mason GA, Wallace KR, Waltron M (1995) Control of wound infection in a thoracic surgery unit. *Lancet* **ii** 786–794.

Chow TT, Yang XY (2004) Ventilation performance in operating theatres against airborne infection; review of research activities and practical guidance. *Journal of Hospital Infection* **56**: 85–92.

Coello R, Charlett A, Wilson J, Pearson A, Borriello P (2005) Adverse impact of surgical site infections in English hospitals. *Journal of Hospital Infection* **60**: 93–103.

Garibaldi RA, Cushing D, Lerer T (1991) Predictors of intra-operative acquired surgical wound infections. *Journal of Hospital Infection* **18**: S1.

Garner S, Gilmore D, Graff L, et al. (2003) *Under Scrutiny – Are You At Risk? Making Sense of New EU Regulations in Medical Devices.* Case Study EN13795. Report from an independent working group. Hsdcommunications, Herts: Rickmansworth.

Garner S, Graff L, Line S, et al. (2002) *Considering the Consequences: An Evaluation of Infection Risk When Choosing Surgical Gowns and Drapes in Today's NHS.* Report from an independent working group. Hsdcommunications, Herts, Rickmansworth.

Graff L, Wigglesworth N, Rose D, et al. (2001) *Surgical Drapes and Gowns in Today's NHS. Moving Forward From Traditional Textiles.* Report from an independent multi-disciplinary working group. Hsdcommunications, Herts: Rickmansworth.

Hedderwick SA, McNeill SA, Lyons KJ, Kaufman CA (2000) Pathogenic organisms associated with artificial fingernails worn by healthcare workers. *Infection Control and Hospital Epidemiology* **21**: 505–509.

Hoffman PN, Bradley CR, Ayliffe GAT (2004) *Disinfection in Healthcare* (3rd edn), Oxford: Blackwell Publishing.

Hoffman PN, Williams J, Stacey A, et al. (2002) Microbiological commissioning and monitoring of operating theatre suites. *Journal of Hospital Infection* **52** (1): 1–28.

Cheswork T, Humphries, H (2002) Operating theatre ventilation standards and the risk of postoperative infection. *Journal of Hospital Infection* **50** (2): 85–90.

Humphries H, Russell AJ, Marshall RJ, Ricketts VE, Reeves DS (1991) The effect of surgical theatre head-gear on air bacterial counts. *Journal of Hospital Infection* **19**: 175–180.

Humphries H, Stacey AR, Taylor EW (1995) Survey of theatres in Great Britain and Ireland. *Journal of Hospital Infection* **30** (4): 245–252.

Leaper DJ (1995) Risk factors for surgical infection. *Journal of Hospital Infection* 1995 **30**: 127–139.

Mangram AJ, Horan TC, Pearson ML, et al. (1999) Guideline for prevention of surgical site infection. *Infection Control and Epidemiology* **20** (4): 247–277.

Medical Devices Agency (1998) *The Validation and Periodic Testing of Benchtop Vacuum Steam Sterilizers.* MDA DB 9804.

Medical Devices Agency (2000) *Single-use Medical Devices: Implications and Consequences of Reuse.* MDA DB2000(04).

Medical Devices Agency (2002) *Benchtop Steam Sterilizers – Guidance on Purchase, Operation and Maintenance.* MDA DB 2002(06).

Medical Devices Agency (2002A) *Steam Penetration Tests in Vacuum Benchtop Sterilizers.* MDA SN2002(24).

Medical Devices Agency (2000B) *Safety Notice: Use of Spirit Based Solutions During Surgical Procedures Requiring the Use of Electrosurgical Equipment.* MDA SN20009170. London: Medical Devices Agency.

Mitchell NJ, Hunt S (1991) Surgical face masks in modern operating rooms – a costly and unnecessary ritual? *Journal of Hospital Infection* 1991 **18**: 239–242.

National Decontamination Training Programme (2004) http://decontamination-training.nhsestates.gov.uk.

NHS Estates (2003) A guide to the decontamination of reusable surgical instruments. http://www.decontamination.nhsestates.gov.uk/downloads/decontam_guide.pdf.

NHS Estates 2002. *Infection Control in the Built Environment.* London: The Stationery Office. ISBN 0-11-322086-3. Also available on the NHS Estates website.

NHS Estates Health Building Notes HBN 26 (2005). NHS website.

NHS Estates *Primary and Social Care Premises – Planning and design guidance. Specialist treatment spaces.* NHS Estates web site. http://primarycare.nhsestates. gov.uk.

NHS Estates. Health Technical Memorandum 2025:Ventilation in Healthcare Premises. 1994. London: HMSO.

Osman C (2000) Asepsis and aseptic practices in the operating room. *Infection Control Today.* http://www.infectioncontroltoday.com/articles/071best.html.

Plowman R, Graves N, Griffin MA, et al. (2001) The rate and cost of hospital acquired infections occurring in patients admitted to selected specialties of a district general hospital in England and the national burden imposed. *Journal of Hospital Infection* **47**: 198–209.

Pratt RJ, Pellowe C, Loveday HP, et al. (2001) The *epic* project: developing national evidence-based guidelines for preventing healthcare associated infections. Phase 1: guidelines for preventing hospital acquired infections. *Journal of Hospital Infection* 2001 **47**: S47–S67.

Roark J (2003) Guidelines for maintaining the sterile field. *Infection Control Today* **7** (8): 14–16.

Romney MG (2001) Surgical face masks in the operating theatre: re-examining the evidence. *Journal of Hospital Infection* **47**: 251–256.

Smyth ETM, Humphries H, Stacey A, Taylor EW, Hoffman P, Bannister G (2005) Survey of operating theatre ventilation facilities for minimally invasive surgery in Great Britain and Northern Ireland: current practice and considerations for the future. *Journal of Hospital Infection* **61**: 112–122.

Woodhead K, Taylor EW, Bannister G. Chesworth T, Hoffman P, Humphries H (2002) Behaviors and rituals in the operating theatre. *Journal of Hospital Infection* **51** (4): 241–255.

11 The Theatre Environment and Equipment

PARVINDERPAL SAINS

INTRODUCTION

The optimal theatre environment should ensure a user-friendly, efficient, sterile and, above all, a safe setting in which to perform a surgical procedure. In this chapter we will consider the elements that are required for such an environment. Guidelines to the design and construction of theatres for major operations and minor operations are largely the same. The main difference being that due to the nature of major operations, which require general anaesthetics, theatres used for major procedures need to be located near an Intensive Care Unit (ICU) and Accident and Emergency department for the rapid transfer of significantly ill patients. Minor elective procedures performed under local anaesthesia can be carried out in dedicated rooms designed and equipped with the necessary equipment. Most hospitals have these rooms located in Day Surgery Units (DSUs). All hospitals should have a committee of professionals from the various specialties (surgery, anaesthetics, nursing and microbiology) to direct and advise in accordance with Department of Health recommendations for the requirements of a surgical theatre environment.

ORGANISATION

Antisepsis in the minor operating theatre is just as important an issue as in the main theatre environment. Clean and dirty streams of traffic should be separated. This can be achieved by the implementation of various zones: a dirty zone forming the disposal area, an aseptic zone where the operative procedure takes place, a clean zone consisting of the scrub room, exit lobby and sterile store, and reception zone where patients are first received. The clean zone should include adequate storage room for general supplies and equipment as well as rest and refreshment facilities for staff. Staff within the

Minor Surgical Procedures for Nurses and Allied Healthcare Professionals. Edited by Shirley Martin.
© 2007 John Wiley & Sons Limited

areas should be able to move freely from one clean area to another without having to negotiate unprotected areas.

The construction of the theatre and the finishes within it should be of a very high standard so as to maintain cleanliness. This includes the provision of smooth, washable surfaces with minimisation of areas which are prone to dust collection, such as the joins between walls, floors and ceilings. The walls should be surfaced with an impervious semi-matt surface with a laminated plastic finish (vinyl paint or epoxy resin paint). Wall colours should be chosen so that they are not tiring to the eye, for example, pale blue or green. Floor coverings should be impervious such as antistatic rubber, vinyl, or terrazzo tiling.

OTHER CONSIDERATIONS

AIR FLOW

The maintenance of directional or laminar air flow helps to provide a minimally contaminated environment at the operating table. This flow may be vertical or horizontal with the air being pumped into the room without returning to the operating room. Most theatres have 20-40 air changes per hour.

TEMPERATURE AND HUMIDITY

Adequate temperature and humidity control also help to maintain infection control. A steady level of both is also desirable for comfort. The usual temperature in theatres is 20–22°C (68–71°F). Control of the temperature and humidity should be integral to the air-conditioning system.

THEATRE FURNITURE

The basic furniture and equipment required for a minor operating list includes:

theatre lighting;
operating table;
electrosurgical equipment;
instrument trolleys;
stools for sitting.

THEATRE LIGHTING

Good lighting of the operative field is essential to adequate surgical access, even with minor procedures.

Usually, the artificial light in theatres makes daylight unnecessary, but the complete absence of windows is psychologically disadvantageous to staff. If windows are fitted, they should be small to minimise solar heat gain or loss and to facilitate heating and ventilation control.

General lighting is achieved by fluorescent tubes or filament lamps. These should be mounted in ceiling recesses and provide even glare-free illumination. For the actual operative field area, shadow-less illumination is vital and can be achieved either by the use of a single light (Figure 11.1) or several lights directed from different angles if required.

There are various types of shadow-less light fittings:

- Multi-reflector fittings – these have six to nine separate lamps with special reflectors. Focusing of light is achieved by a knob fixed to the fitting.
- Metal reflector fittings – the reflector consists of a concave highly polished metal surface made from a single sheet or having many facets.
- Scialytic fittings – these consist of an optical lens surrounded by a single lamp from which light rays are projected on to a circle of mirrors focusing light on the operating area with the aid of a lamp holder.

The light fittings may be suspended from the ceiling or free standing. Either should allow enough manoeuvrability to provide a multiplicity of positions. The fittings should be easily cleaned with minimum maintenance. Ideally the control panel for the lights should be separate to the lights and a sterile handle should be used to position the light during a procedure.

The stability and mobility of the light fittings should be checked regularly as well as making sure that the fittings are clean and dust free. All bulbs and switches should be checked and maintained daily.

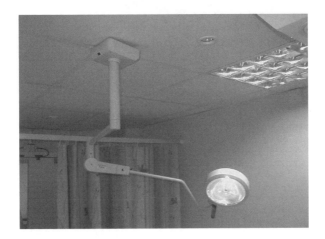

Figure 11.1 Single operating light.

OPERATING TABLE

As in all types of surgery, the correct positioning of the patient in minor surgery is vital for adequate access to the operative site, patient comfort, and safety. Many minor procedures can be carried out on trolleys but it is recommended that a dedicated operating table is used. This can be adjusted, either manually or electronically, to give a variety of positions and also adapted for specific procedures.

Operating tables (Figure 11.2) need to be heavy and stable, easily adjustable, manoeuvrable and comfortable for the patient. Features of a mobile operating table include: brakes, raising and lowering mechanism, lateral tilting mechanism, Trendelenburg/reverse tilting mechanism adjustable head and foot sections, antistatic mattress, rotating table top, chair/sitting mechanism. Before each use of the operating table, the integrity of the antistatic mattress should be checked as well as the correct working of all mechanisms likely to be used to position the patient adequately. The table must also be clean and dust free. It is recommended that the table, accessories (eg arm boards) and mattress should be cleaned with detergent and warm water after each use.

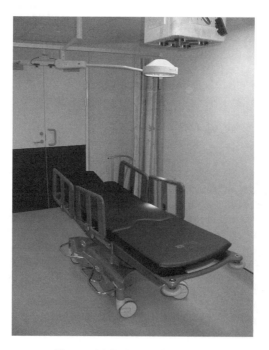

Figure 11.2 Operating table.

ELECTROSURGICAL DIATHERMY UNITS

The use of diathermy units is limited in minor surgery. However, they are occasionally required when haemostasis cannot be achieved by other methods. The use of diathermy is discussed further in Chapter 16.

All electrosurgical units should be regularly maintained with readily available operating manuals. The units should be clean and dust free with alarm systems, plugs and leads checked prior to the patient's arrival. The unit should be plugged in, with foot pedals and connections correctly attached and positioned. Power settings should be checked by the operator.

TROLLEYS AND SEATS

All other furniture should be clean, dust free and should be cleaned between every procedure with detergent and water. Trolleys should be made of stainless steel, aluminum or steel covered nylon. They should be abrasion- and scratch-free. Stool seats (Figure 11.3) should be covered with an anti-static material with particular attention paid to the wheel and positioning mechanisms.

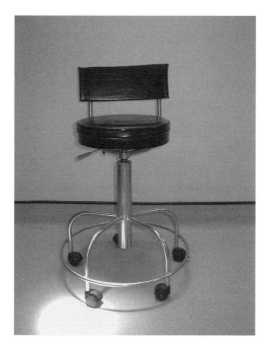

Figure 11.3 Theatre stool.

12 Recognising Skin Lesions

JULIA SCHOFIELD

INTRODUCTION

It is important to have some basic knowledge and understanding of types of skin lesions to ensure that the appropriate surgical procedure is performed when removing a skin lesion. This chapter will look at the commoner skin lesions and aim to provide tips about their recognition.

Common skin lesions are derived from the structures within normal skin (Figure 12.1). It is helpful to understand and relate the structure of the skin to common skin lesions. Figure 12.1 shows the epidermis and the dermis beneath. The appearance of the skin lesion is determined by the type of cells or tissue and the site from which it is derived.

EPIDERMAL LESIONS

The epidermis comprises keratinocytes and melanocytes and the commonest epidermal lesions will be derived from these cell types.

Keratinocytes

Layers of keratinocytes make up most of the epidermis and form the uppermost external waterproof protective layer of the skin. Lesions derived from epidermal keratinocytes will therefore usually be crusty, scaly, rough and superficial. This change is known as keratotic. Such lesions will give the impression of being able to be easily lifted off the skin. An example of this is a seborrhoeic keratosis. These are benign skin lesions and are shown in Figure 12.2 below including a diagrammatic representation.

Other examples of keratotic lesions derived from the keratinocytes of the epidermis include solar keratoses, squamous cell carcinoma and Bowen's disease (intraepidermal squamous cell carcinoma).

Minor Surgical Procedures for Nurses and Allied Healthcare Professionals. Edited by Shirley Martin.
© 2007 John Wiley & Sons Limited

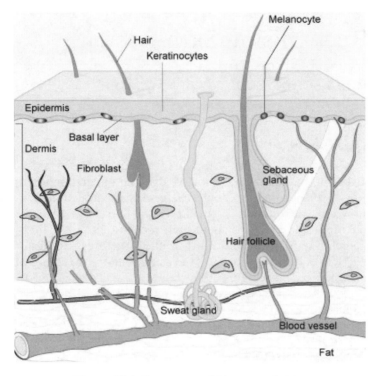

Figure 12.1 Structures within normal skin.

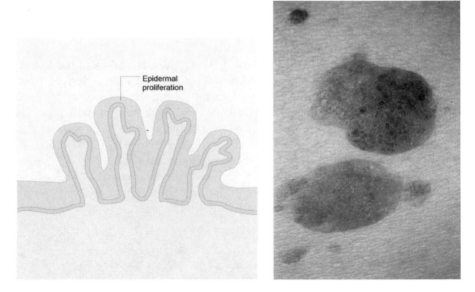

Figure 12.2 Seborrhoeic keratosis.

Melanocytic lesions

Melanocytic lesions are derived from melanocytes in the basal layer of the epidermis and benign proliferations of melanocytes are called melanocytic naevi. Melanocytes are pigmented and so most melanocytic lesions will be pigmented. Melanocytic lesions commonly develop in childhood and early adult life and evolve as shown in Figures 12.3 to 12.5 below.

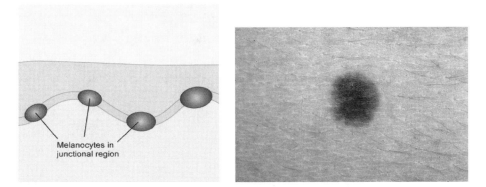

Figure 12.3 Junctional melanocytic naevus: proliferation of melanocytes at the basal/junctional layer results in a flat deeply pigmented lesion.

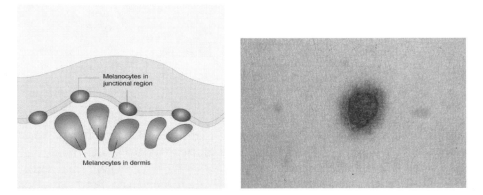

Figure 12.4 Compound melanocytic naevus: here some of the proliferating melanocytes have dropped into the dermis resulting in the overlying skin becoming raised. The lesion remains pigmented as there is on-going melanocytic activity at the basement layer.

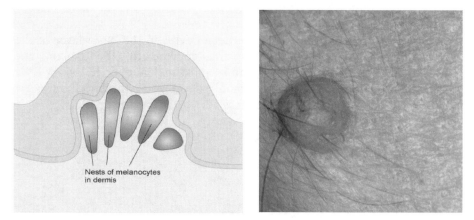

Figure 12.5 Intradermal melanocytic naevus: here most of the melanocytes have dropped into the dermis and the lesion is therefore raised. There is little remaining junctional melanocytic activity and the melanocytes are deeper in the skin. The lesion therefore no longer looks pigmented.

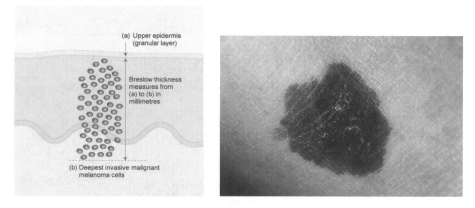

Figure 12.6 Malignant melanoma.

This maturation process can halt at any stage of development of a melanocytic naevus but many will evolve through all three stages as they mature.

In malignant melanoma the melanocytic proliferation is of abnormal malignant melanocytes which invade the underlying dermis. The depth to which the malignant melanocytes invade is called the Breslow thickness and this measurement largely determines the prognosis of malignant melanoma. The smaller the Breslow thickness, the thinner the tumour and the better the prognosis (Figure 12.6).

DERMAL LESIONS

Lesions arising from dermal structures will usually have a smooth normal overlying skin and be elevated. The thickness of the lesion is usually similar to the diameter. The common structures in the dermis that give rise to skin lesions include hair follicles, fibrocytes (which produce fibrous tissue) and blood vessels. The types of lesion produced are shown below.

Related to hair follicles: pilar or epidermoid cyst

These lesions are commonly known as sebaceous cysts but this is inaccurate. True sebaceous cysts are actually extremely rare whilst epidermoid or pilar cysts are quite common (Figure 12.7).

Proliferation of dermal fibrous tissue

Dermatofibromas are formed from a proliferation of fibrous cells within the dermis and are thought to represent an abnormal response to an insect bite. These lesions commonly occur on the lower limb particularly in women and are often itchy. They are very firm nodules and are usually pink but can also be pigmented (Figure 12.8).

Lesions due to blood vessels in the dermis

There are several common lesions related to blood vessels. The commonest is the spider naevus (Figure 12.9). Here, instead of the dermal blood vessel growing parallel to the overlying epidermis, the vessel grows up towards the

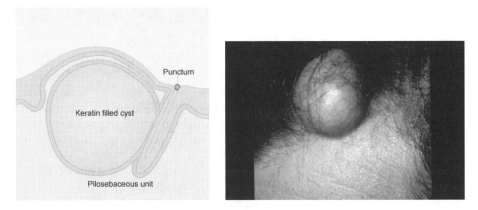

Figure 12.7 Pilar or epidermoid cyst.

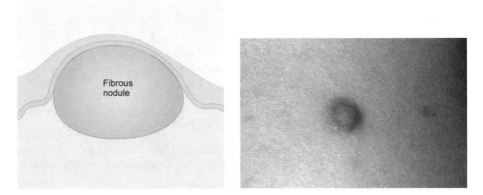

Figure 12.8 Dermatofibroma.

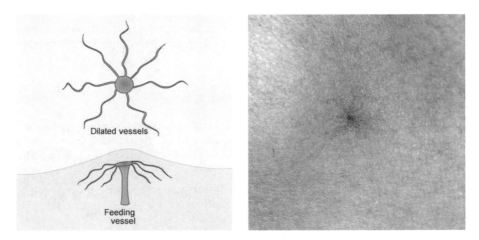

Figure 12.9 Spider naevus.

epidermis (Figure 12.9). These are common in normal individuals but can be seen particularly as a result of excess oestrogens, for example in puberty, pregnancy and in patients taking an oestrogen-containing contraceptive pill.

Pyogenic granulomas occur as a result of over-proliferation of blood vessels. They typically occur on the extremities (usually digits) and often seem to develop following a history of trauma to the affected area. These are very vascular and tend to bleed profusely when knocked (Figure 12.10).

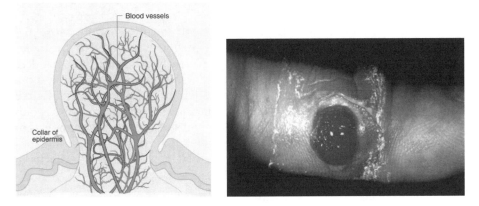

Figure 12.10 Pyogenic granuloma.

WHAT ARE THE COMMON SKIN LESIONS?

When trying to recognise skin lesions it is helpful to know which are the commonest that are encountered during skin surgery. The list below reflects the frequency of skin lesions removed in a twelve month period in Primary Care and gives some idea of the commonest skin lesions that are likely to be encountered by practitioners performing skin surgery.

29% Melanocytic naevus
24% Seborrhoeic keratosis
16% Epidermoid cyst
12% Skin tag
 5% Dermatofibroma
 2% Malignant lesions
12% Other, including pyogenic granuloma.

TIPS FROM THE CLINICAL HISTORY

The clinical history is crucial when trying to identify and treat skin lesions. There will be important clues from the history to help in recognising what the lesion is likely to be. More importantly the history helps to clarify whether a lesion is likely to be benign or malignant. This should enable the diagnosing clinician to decide whether a patient should be advised to have a lesion removed promptly because of suspected malignancy. It is helpful for surgical practitioners to understand the factors that may influence clinical diagnosis and some of these are outlined below.

How old is the patient?

The age of the patient provides us with important information. Most pigmented lesions seen in young adults will be melanocytic. Whilst new moles commonly appear in childhood, puberty and early adult life they are less likely to appear in the fouth or fifth decade. One would therefore be more worried about a malignant melanoma in a patient presenting with a new mole who is 50 years of age rather than 15. In contrast seborrhoeic keratoses commonly appear in the fifth or sixth decade and are the most common skin lesions seen in elderly patients. Skin lesions related to cumulative sun exposure such as non-melanoma skin cancer (see later) are unlikely to occur in young adults but are commoner in the elderly.

Is the lesion changing?

A new or pre-existing skin lesion that is enlarging quickly (over weeks or months) will cause more concern to the diagnosing clinician than a long standing lesion demonstrating a slow change over a long period of time (many years) as the former is more likely to suggest malignant change. The changes that one is particularly concerned about are as follows.

- For suspected malignant melanoma: change in size, shape or colour of a melanocytic lesion.
- For suspected non-melanoma skin cancer: a persistent changing or non-healing lesion over weeks or months, often on skin that is regularly exposed to sunlight.

Remember: most malignant melanomas will be bigger than 7mm in diameter. Melanocytic naevi that are stable and not changing are very unlikely to be malignant.

Is the lesion symptomatic?

Crusting, bleeding and itching are sometimes features of malignant change in skin lesions (particularly melanocytic naevi) but are much less important than a change in size, shape or colour. Studies suggest that itching alone is not usually a sign of malignant change in melanocytic naevi.

Are there any other pointers to skin malignancy?

Skin type is an important factor in relation to skin cancer risk. Those who burn easily being more prone to develop skin cancer than those who tan readily. It is always helpful to get some idea of how much sun exposure patients have had to relate this to whether a diagnosis of skin cancer is likely. Those who have spent many years in sunny climes are much more likely to be at risk of skin cancer. A history of sunburn in childhood is particularly associated with skin cancer risk. A previous history of skin cancer suggests an increased risk in developing other skin cancers.

TIPS FROM THE CLINICAL EXAMINATION

It is helpful to describe a skin lesion using agreed terminology. This can then give clues to the diagnosis. The following terms are typically useful.

- Keratotic means crusty/warty. This suggests a superficial epidermally derived lesion such as a seborrhoeic keratosis or solar keratosis.
- Cyst is a cavity lined with epithelium. The commonest cyst is an epidermoid cyst. These lesions are usually fixed to the skin and there is usually a punctum visible representing a follicular orifice.
- Nodule usually represents dermal pathology. The commonest cause of a firm dermal nodule is a dermatofibroma.

RECOGNISING SKIN LESIONS: SKIN CANCER

No section on skin lesions would be complete without a short overview for practitioners about the common types of skin cancer.

Skin cancer is common. There are around 60000 reported cases of skin cancer per annum in the UK. Skin cancer is divided into two main groups, which are melanoma (mole) skin cancer and non-melanoma skin cancer. Non-melanoma skin cancer is very common and rarely life-threatening whereas malignant melanoma is much less common but more serious.

Non-melanoma skin cancer includes basal cell carcinoma (BCC) and squamous cell carcinoma (SCC) (Figures 12.11 and 12.12). BCC is commoner than SCC. There is a link between long term sun exposure and the development of these types of non-melanoma skin cancer. Both are best treated by surgical excision. BCCs are unlikely to metastasise whereas SCCs sometimes do metastasise.

Whilst malignant melanoma is less common it is a more serious type of skin cancer and early diagnosis is very important in determining cure. The only available successful treatment for malignant melanoma currently is early surgical excision. The outlook is determined by the Breslow thickness at the time of presentation (see page 140). Features suggesting the development of malignant melanoma include change in size, shape or colour of existing moles or a new mole growing over a period of weeks or months (Figure 12.13).

RECOGNISING SKIN LESIONS: WHY BOTHER?

Correct diagnosis = correct surgical procedure
Incorrect diagnosis = incorrect surgical procedure

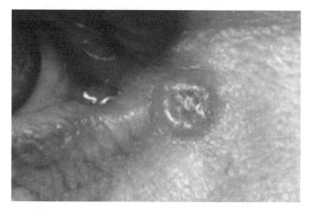

Figure 12.11 Basal cell carcinoma.

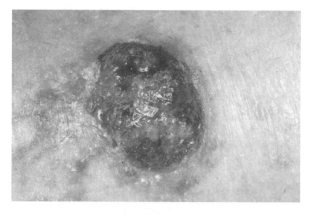

Figure 12.12 Squamous cell carcinoma.

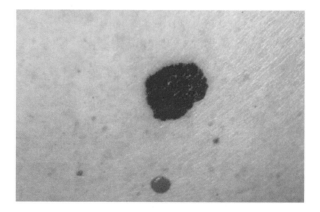

Figure 12.13 Malignant melanoma.

A common example of an inappropriate surgical procedure is the removal of a seborrhoeic keratosis by ellipse excision. The patient has a resultant linear sutured scar. If the surgical removal of a seborrhoeic keratosis is indicated the correct surgical procedure is curettage and cautery. The following are examples of appropriate surgical procedures.

- Seborrhoeic keratosis: curettage and cautery.
- Skin tags: snip excision.
- Intradermal melanocytic naevus: shave excision.
- Changing melanocytic naevus: ellipse excision with 2 mm margin.

The surgical practitioner should not be expected to be an expert diagnostician of skin lesions. However, the practitioner has a responsibility to feel comfortable that the procedure they are performing is appropriate for the skin lesion and that the surgery is being undertaken in a timely fashion. The referring diagnostician should document the differential diagnosis and the surgical procedure requested should be appropriate to the proposed diagnosis. Hopefully this chapter has provided some useful background to support this approach.

© Schofield and Kneebone. *Skin Lesions. A practice guide to diagnosis management and minor surgery. Second edition.*

13 Basic Anatomy and Techniques of Excising Skin Lesions

GREGORY THOMAS AND SANJAY PURKAYASTHA
(Ilustrations by Olivia Thomas)

INTRODUCTION

Health problems that require minor surgical intervention are very common. These cause patients a great deal of distress, and also put a lot of pressure on already over-stretched hospital resources. With the changes currently being implemented to doctors' working hours and training programmes, it has become necessary to develop the role of surgical practitioner. These are healthcare workers with sufficient training for them to undertake much of this work. In centres all over the UK there are now nurse practitioners who have developed the necessary skills for them to perform minor surgical procedures and lead their own outpatient clinics. The role of the surgical practitioner will be an increasingly important one in the NHS of tomorrow.

THE STRUCTURE OF SKIN

The skin is composed of three layers:

- epidermis;
- dermis;
- hypodermis or subcutaneous tissue.

The epidermal layer is avascular, and is composed of stratified squamous epithelial cells. It is around 0.04 to 0.4 mm thick. It is thicker in certain parts of the body, such as soles of the feet or palms of the hands.

The dermis is a vascular layer. It contains blood vessels, which arise from a deeper vascular plexus, nerves, sweat glands and lymphatic vessels. It is around 0.5 to 2.5 mm thick.

Minor Surgical Procedures for Nurses and Allied Healthcare Professionals. Edited by Shirley Martin.
© 2007 John Wiley & Sons Limited

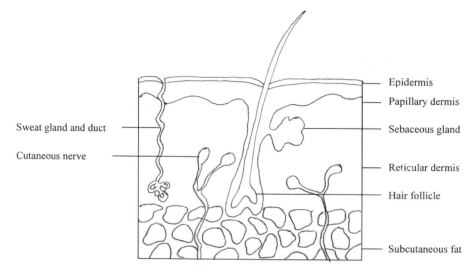

Figure 13.1 Cross section of skin.

SOME COMMON BENIGN SKIN LESIONS

SKIN TAGS

These are benign tumours of the epidermis. They are small growths, with a pedunculated shape. They consist of a loose connective tissue core surrounded by epidermis and can sometimes be pigmented. They are common and are most usually seen in the middle aged to elderly age group. They are thought to arise from areas where skin surfaces rub together, and chronic irritation takes place. Examples of such areas are the axilla, groin and neck.

BENIGN PIGMENTED NAEVI

These are formed by an increased focal population of melanocytes (pigment containing cells of the skin). They can occur at various levels in the skin. They occur at any age, but are more commonly seen in the second decade of life. They are very common, and at least one will be present in over 95% of the population. They can sometimes be confused with malignant melanomas. These are malignant tumours of melanocyte cells, and can have a very poor prognosis if left untreated. However, naevi are usually benign before puberty.

Certain characteristics can be looked for in a lesion that may arouse suspicion of malignancy, these are:

- Change in size
- Change in shape
- Change in colour
- Mild itching

- Asymmetrical
- Irregular border
- Irregular colour

- Diameter >7 mm
- Inflammation around lesion
- Bleeding

SEBACEOUS CYSTS

These are also known as pilar or epidermal cysts. They consist of a collection of keratin and keratin breakdown products surrounded by a wall of stratified squamous keratinising epithelium. They are very common. They tend to be found on areas that have hair follicles. The most common site is the scalp. Sebaceous cysts are usually solitary, but can be found in small clusters. They are discrete masses, found in the deeper layers of the skin, but are mobile over the deeper structures. Often they will have a central overlying punctum. It is possible for these lesions to become infected, in which case they will require incision and drainage.

LIPOMA

A benign tumour of fat, or adipose tissue. When seen on the skin, these lesions usually arise from the subcutaneous layer of fat. They can appear at any stage of life, but are more commonly seen in middle age. They are usually seen on the head, neck, abdomen and thighs, but can appear anywhere there is adipose tissue. They are usually asymptomatic, but can cause distress if they are impinging on surrounding structures. Care should be taken when planning the excision of the larger ones since they can become very closely related to or surround nearby structures such as nerves and blood vessels.

GANGLION

This is a small tense cyst that contains a viscous jelly-like material. They are associated with joints and tendon sheaths. They often occur at the wrist, but may also be seen at the hands and feet. They are thought to be caused by the presence of synovium outside a joint. They are usually asymptomatic, presenting only a cosmetic problem. If not completely removed during surgery, they tend to re-occur.

KELOID SCAR

This is an overgrowth of scar tissue that extends beyond the boundaries of the original scar. They are more common in the Afro-Caribbean and oriental ethnic groups. Their removal can be very problematic.

PLANNING AND PREPARING THE PROCEDURE

THE DIAGNOSIS

There should always be a referral clinic letter from a senior surgeon who has reviewed this patient. This should contain a working diagnosis of the lesion in question, or at the very least a differential diagnosis to work with. The letter should also contain the suggested management plan.

THE NECESSITY OF THE PROCEDURE

Sound reasons for performing a procedure would be:

- if the lesion is symptomatic;
- if it is becoming subjected to repeated trauma;
- if there is a strong cosmetic argument;
- if there is a suspicion that the lesion may be malignant.

THE COSMETIC EFFECT OF THE PROCEDURE

Any form of incision, providing the dermo-epidermal junction is penetrated, will leave some form of a scar. However, certain measures can be taken to minimise the effect of this.

The skin is composed of many natural tension lines, or Langer's lines. These show the 'grain' of the skin. They lie at right angles to the direction of contraction of the underlying muscle fibres, but will be arranged in a parallel fashion around the connective tissue dermal collagen bundles. These lines can often be seen on the face and neck as wrinkle or laughter lines. On the rest of the body they tend to follow a transverse pattern. Figure 13.2 illustrates their general arrangement.

A surgical incision placed along one of these lines will heal into a thin, strong and cosmetically pleasing scar, with minimal contracture occurring. If, however, the incision is placed across one of these lines then a weaker, wider scar is produced with a greater chance of a contracture occurring.

As with Langer's lines, joint crease lines should also be followed when an incision is made, otherwise the above problems will occur. Here, contractures of the skin may have a damaging effect on the function of the underlying joint.

Equally, if the lesion is present on the face, neck or on the hands there needs to be a greater consideration of the resulting cosmetic effect. Lesions on the hands, neck and face should be referred to a senior surgeon. Questions to consider would be the size of the scar likely to be left afterwards and the likelihood of a contracture? As small an incision as possible is desired if the lesion is in these areas.

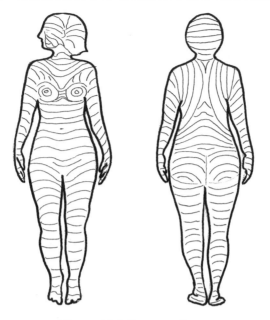

Figure 13.2 Langer's lines.

Accurate, durable preoperative skin marking, that will withstand the preoperative skin preparation, is vital. This allows the planned incision to be marked out, and helps to avoid any confusion or mistakes during the procedure.

Too much tension across a wound when closing, will lead to sub-optimal healing and development of a larger scar.

Some sutures can trigger a larger inflammatory effect than others. If the sutures are left in too long or too big a choice of suture is made, then a 'laddering effect' can occur.

DAMAGE TO SURROUNDING STRUCTURES

It is possible that damage may be caused to surrounding structures. These can be classified into superficial and deeper structures.

- Superficial structures – surrounding skin, hair follicles, sebaceous glands.
- Deeper structures – blood vessels, nerves and tendons.

WOUND INFECTION

Infection is a risk with any surgical incision or procedure. This can be minimised by a careful patient preparation, rigorous sterile technique during the procedure, good wound closure and the possible use of perioperative antibiotics.

PATIENT PREPARATION

It is important that the skin is prepared. Shaving, if required, needs to be done immediately before the procedure, otherwise the surrounding hair needs to be clipped. A chlorhexidine, or iodine containing solution should be used to clean the skin. This should be applied in a circular fashion, moving away from the area of planned incision. Sterile drapes should then be placed over the area, so that a sterile field is created around the site of the proposed procedure.

Warfarin may be stopped prior to the procedure. However the risks of doing this should be considered and if in doubt the advice of a senior doctor should be sought.

If the patient is diabetic, their blood sugar control should be optimised prior to surgery, and the patient should be put first on the operating list.

CONSENT

Informed consent is covered in detail in chapter 5. The patient should be made fully aware of the possibility of scars, wound complications, damage to surrounding structures and recurrence of disease.

HAZARDOUS SITES

As mentioned earlier, special consideration needs to be given to the cosmetic implications when removing skin lesions from the face, neck and hands. There are certain areas of the body that have a greater proportion of potentially hazardous structures than other areas. These are the face, neck, axillae, antecubital fossae, groin and popliteal spaces. These areas all contain large blood vessels and nerves that lie close to the surface, and as such are more easily damaged. Any procedure in these areas should be referred to an experienced surgeon.

REMOVAL OF A SEBACEOUS CYST

- The cyst should be thoroughly examined before the procedure, so that an accurate size of the lesion can be deduced. It is sometimes possible to underestimate the size of some sebaceous cysts, especially those on the back.
- An elliptical incision is required. This should be narrow, and its ideal length should be around 3 to 4 times its width. It should directly overlie the cyst, as shown in Figure 13.3. At least 0.5 cm of tissue needs to be included beyond the cyst.

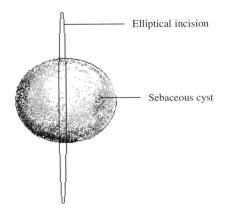

Elliptical incision

Sebaceous cyst

Figure 13.3 Incision around sebaceous cyst.

- Infiltrate the area with local anaesthetic.
- Make the incision, and then dissect around the cyst down to the subcutaneous layer, trying to avoid rupturing the cyst if possible. As the tissue around the cyst is dissected, the cyst should be held in non-traumatising forceps, so that an element of tension is applied.
- The cyst can then be removed. It is important to remove the cyst in its entirety, including its capsule; otherwise there is a risk of it re-occurring.
- When closing the incision, the dermis and resulting space should be closed first. This can be done with absorbable interrupted sutures of 4-0 or 5-0.
- The epidermis should then be closed with 5-0 absorbable, undyed, braided or non-braided sutures in a sub-cuticular continuous or interrupted fashion. The wound can be reinforced with steri-strips if required.
- A semi-occlusive dressing should be applied over the wound for 24–48 hours. Give the patient instructions to keep the wound dry for this period and to avoid any excessive movement to this area.
- As with all excisions, the tissue excised needs to be sent for histological examination. The results of this will need to be followed up and the patient will need to be informed.

REMOVAL OF A SMALL SUPERFICIAL SKIN LIPOMA

- Small superficial lipomata can easily be removed under local anaesthetic.
- Examine the lipoma first, making sure it is not deeply tethered (eg to underlying muscular layers or to a body cavity) and that it is located solely in a superficial plane, and is freely mobile. Sometimes, lipomata may be located below the deep facial layer, these and the larger ones need to be referred to a senior surgeon for removal.

Incision:

2/3 diameter of lesion

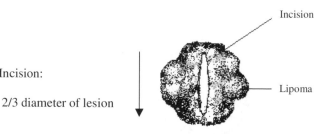

Figure 13.4 Incision for removal of lipoma.

- After the area has been anaesthetised, a linear incision should be made, over the lipoma. If the lipoma is large, then an elliptical incision may be used. If so, this ellipse's length should be 3 to 4 times greater than its width. The length of the ellipse need only be two thirds of the length of its underlying lesion (Figure 13.4).
- The lipoma can be easily distinguished from the surrounding subcutaneous fat. It should be well defined and enclosed in a fine capsule.
- Once visualised, the lipoma should be 'shelled-out' by blunt dissection, using your finger or a pair of scissors.
- Sometimes a lipoma may have an underlying blood vessel. There may be a small amount of bleeding occurring here. If this occurs, applying pressure using a piece of gauze should be sufficient to achieve haemostasis. If this is not sufficient, diathermy can be used, and if this is not successful the vessel responsible will need to be tied off.
- The wound should then be closed, as described above, with the same post-op management plan.

REMOVAL OF A SIMPLE BENIGN NAEVUS

- These lesions can be removed by a simple elliptical excision. If there is any doubt about the benign nature of the lesion, it should be referred to a senior surgeon for urgent review.
- An elliptical incision should be made around the lesion, in the same proportions explained above. An excision margin of a couple of millimetres should be left around the lesion (Figure 13.5).

Once excised the wound should be closed, as explained above. The tissue should be sent for histology and followed up.

REMOVAL OF A SKIN TAG

- This can be achieved by a technique know as 'snip excision'. This technique can also be used for narrow necked fibro-epithelial polyps.

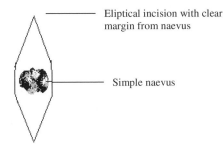

Eliptical incision with clear margin from naevus

Simple naevus

Figure 13.5 Diagram showing removal of a simple benign naevus.

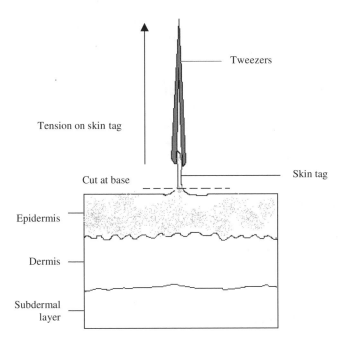

Tweezers

Tension on skin tag

Skin tag

Cut at base

Epidermis

Dermis

Subdermal layer

Figure 13.6 A snip excision.

- The area in question should first be infiltrated with local anaesthetic.
- The lesion is held up by a pair of forceps, and the neck of the lesion is cut with a sharp pair of scissors (Figure 13.6).
- There is often a small amount of bleeding following this incision. This can usually be controlled by applying pressure for a few minutes. Sometimes diathermy may be needed to achieve haemostasis.
- Alternatively, skin tags can be removed by shaving.

REMOVAL OF SEBORRHOIC KERATOSES

- Seborrhoic keratoses can be removed using a technique called curettage. This technique is also applicable to the removal of warts.
- Firstly, the area is infiltrated with local anaesthetic.
- Then a curette is dragged across the lesion, this should remove it. It is important that the plane that the curette moves in is parallel to the plane of the skin surface. This is because the curette is very sharp, and quite liable to dig deeper into the skin, and take a bite out of the dermal layer (Figure 13.7).
- It is also possible to shave off these lesions. Here, the area in question is first anaesthetised, and then a sharp shaving razor is dragged over the lesion.
- There may be a small amount of oozing of blood, or even frank bleeding. Pressure over the area is usually sufficient to control this. Occasionally diathermy may be required for haemostasis.

REMOVAL OF A SIMPLE GANGLION

- Those ganglia that are located on the limbs, toes and fingers are usually suitable for this method of removal. If the ganglion is located over the ventral aspect of the wrist it is wise to refer this patient on for review by a senior surgeon, since it is likely to be in very close proximity to various tendons, nerves and blood vessels.
- Infiltrate the ganglion with local anaesthetic.
- Using a large needle (21G) and syringe, drain the ganglion via aspiration.
- A sclerosing agent (sodium tetradecyl, STD 3% w/v) should then be injected into the ganglion space.
- A gauze pressure dressing should be applied over the top of it.

REMOVAL OF AN INGROWN TOENAIL (ONYCHOCRYPTOSIS)

- For total excision, or avulsion, of the nail, position the patient in the supine position, and prepare the distal part of the affected foot.
- Apply a double rubber band tourniquet around the proximal phalanx of the affected toe to create an avascular field. This should be removed as soon as possible afterwards to reduce the risk of digital ischaemia.
- Apply a digital nerve block to the digit using local anaesthetic, and allow time for this to work.
- Insert a straight haemostat directly under the nail, in the area of inflammation. Push the instrument in until it reaches the lunula (distal border of the nail matrix).

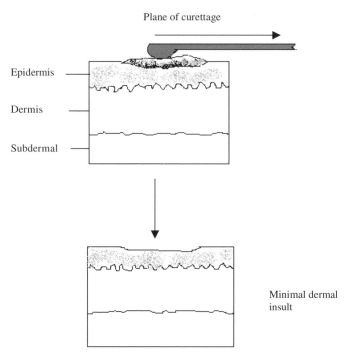

Figure 13.7 Seborrhoic curettage.

- Roll the instrument and nail towards the opposite side for complete avulsion of the nail. It is important to ensure that all nail fragments are removed.
- Ensure all the granulation tissue is removed, this may be achieved with electrocautery or with a currette.
- Cover the area with antibiotic ointment, and apply a sterile dressing. Antibiotic ointment should be applied daily until healing is complete. The patient should be told to refrain from strenuous exercise for at least one week.
- If only a partial excision of nail and matrix is required, only the affected part of the nail is removed.
- The lateral affected part of the nail is excised using scalpel or nail splitter, and then extracted using a haemostat or forceps.
- It is important to ensure that the underlying matrix, necrotic tissue and granulation tissue are removed.
- The postoperative instructions are the same as above

REMOVAL OF A KELOID SCAR

- Surgical excision alone of these scars will almost certainly lead to a recurrence.
- Intra-lesion corticosteroid injection has been proved to be beneficial. Triamcinolone acetonide is the corticosteroid of choice here.
- This should be mixed with lignocaine, and infiltrated into the lesion. This will often need to be repeated over a period of time.
- The use of cryosurgery to the lesion beforehand has been shown to enhance the effects of the corticosteroid. Liquid nitrogen is applied for a period of 5–15 seconds, then left for 15 minutes, at which point the corticosteroids can be given.
- Combinations of corticosteroids and surgery and radiotherapy have also been shown to be beneficial.

FURTHER READING

English RS, Shenefelt PD (1999). Keloids and hypertrophic scars. *Dermatologic Surgery* **25** (8).

Malcolm (1999) Sebaceous cysts. *Practitioner* **243** (1596): 226.

Martin S (2002) Developing the nurse practitioner's role in minor surgery. *Nursing Times* **98** (33).

Price CJ, Sinclair R (2001) *Minor Surgery*. Oxford: Health Press.

Russell RC, Williams NS, Bulstrode CJ (2004) *Bailey & Love's Short Practice of Surgery*, 24th edn. London: Arnold.

Sodera VK (1994) *Minor Surgery in Practice*. Cambridge: Cambridge University Press.

Skandalakis JE, Skandalakis PN, Skandalakis LJ (2000) *Surgical Anatomy and Technique. A Pocket Manual*, 2nd edn. New York: Springer.

Tatla T, Laffarty K (2002) Making your mark again in surgery. *Annals of the Royal College of Surgeons of England* **84** (2): 129–130.

Zuber TJ (2002) Ingrown toenail removal. *American Family Physician* **65** (12).

14 Local Anaesthesia for Minor Operative Procedures

DAVID LOMAX AND KAUSI RAO

With the modernisation of the NHS, the number of patients being treated as day cases is increasing. Non-medical practitioners and other allied health professionals are now performing minor procedures and part of their training must include the safe use of local anaesthesia. In the day care setting, local anaesthesia offers the advantage of quicker recovery and discharge. Local anaesthetics eliminate pain without inducing unconsciousness and so allow for surgery to take place without the use of sedative drugs. They produce reversible conduction blockade of nerve impulses in a unique way.

MECHANISM OF ACTION

Transmission of an impulse along a nerve depends upon the electrical gradient across the nerve membrane. The gradient is determined by the movement of sodium (Na^+) and potassium (K^+) ions across this membrane. An impulse is transmitted along a nerve by Na^+ ions migrating from outside the lipid nerve membrane to within. This is called depolarisation. This is followed by repolarisation, when K^+ ions move in the opposite direction.

Local anaesthetics work by preventing the migration of ions across nerve membranes thus blocking membrane depolarisation. They are 'membrane stabilisers'.

Another mechanism of action is by 'membrane expansion'. This is where the drug dissolves into the phospholipid membrane of the nerve causing swelling of the Na^+ channel/lipoprotein matrix resulting in its inactivation.

PREPARATIONS OF LOCAL ANAESTHETICS

Local anaesthetics are formulated as water-soluble salts. The solutions are usually acidic. These preparations may also contain preservatives, which helps to maintain the stability of the solution, while fungicides (thymol), prevent the growth of contaminating fungi.

Minor Surgical Procedures for Nurses and Allied Healthcare Professionals. Edited by Shirley Martin.
© 2007 John Wiley & Sons Limited

Vasopressors may be used. Adrenaline 1:200000 or felypressin (a synthetic derivative of vasopressin with no antidiuretic effect) is added to some local anaesthetic solutions to slow down absorption from the site of injection and to prolong the duration of action. They decrease the bleeding and increase the total volume and dose that can be given to the patient.

Vasopressors are contraindicated for infiltration around any 'end organs' such as fingers or toes. They should also not be used when performing intravenous regional anaesthesia such as a Bier's block.

Glucose at 80mg/ml may be added to bupivacaine to make a 'heavy' solution. This means that it is hyperbaric as compared to cerebrospinal fluid and only has use in 'spinal' anaesthesia.

STRUCTURE ACTIVITY RELATIONSHIPS

Local anaesthetics consist of a lipophilic aromatic group (essential for anaesthetic activity), an intermediate ester (—CO.O—) or amide (—NH.CO—) chain, and a hydrophilic secondary or tertiary amine group. The intermediate chain allows local anaesthetics to be classified as esters or amides.

Ester local anaesthetics include:

- Cocaine
- Procaine
- Cheoroprocaine
- Amethocaine.

Amide local anaesthetics are:

- Lignocaine
- Prilocaine
- Bupivacaine
- Ropivacaine.

The differences between ester and amide local anaesthetics relate to the site of metabolism and the potential for producing allergic reactions.

Esters are relatively unstable in solution, and are rapidly hydrolysed in the body by plasma cholinesterase, as well as some other esterases. By contrast, amides are relatively stable in solution and are slowly broken down by amidases in the liver (Figure 14.1). Hypersensitivity reactions to amide local anaesthetics are very rare.

PHYSICOCHEMICAL CHARACTERISTICS

The individual structures confer different physicochemical and clinical characteristics.

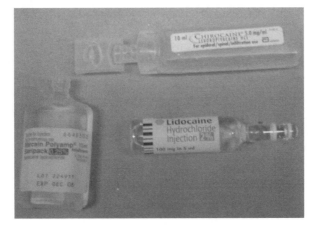

Figure 14.1 Local anaesthetics.

POTENCY

This is correlated to lipid solubility so that increased lipid solubility increases the drug's ability to penetrate the lipid cell membrane and hence increases its potency.

DURATION OF ACTION

This is associated with the extent of protein binding. Sodium channels are formed from large protein molecules and local anaesthetics with longer durations of action bind to these proteins for longer periods.

ONSET OF ACTION

The speed of onset of local anaesthesia depends upon the amount of unionised form of the drug that presents itself to the nerve membrane. This depends on its pKa value. Local anaesthetics are weak bases (as opposed to acids) and exist mainly in the ionised form at a normal pH.

Those with a high pKa have a greater fraction present in the ionised form, which is unable to penetrate the phospholipid membrane, resulting in a slow onset of action. Conversely, a low pKa reflects a higher fraction in the unionised form and therefore a faster onset of action because more is available to cross the phospholipid membrane.

VASOMOTOR EFFECTS

The intrinsic vasodilator activity varies between drugs and influences potency and duration of action. Local anaesthetics cause vasodilatation in low concentration and vasoconstriction at higher concentrations. However, cocaine has solely vasoconstrictor actions by inhibiting neuronal uptake of catecholamines and inhibiting monoamine oxidase.

The total dose and concentration of local anaesthetic given will also have an effect on the above as will other clinical factors.

CLINICAL FACTORS AFFECTING THE ACTION OF LOCAL ANAESTHETICS

DOSE

Increasing the dose will shorten its onset time and increase the duration of block.

VOLUME

Increasing the volume usually means an increased dose and will increase the duration of block.

SITE OF INJECTION

Larger nerves such as motor nerves take longer to be blocked by local anaesthetics and duration of action will be shortened in a more vascular area. The quickest onset of action is probably skin anaesthesia following dermal infiltration and the slowest, epidural anaesthesia.

INFECTED TISSUE

Local anaesthetics are generally ineffective when used to anaesthetise infected tissue. The acidic environment reduces the un-ionised fraction of drug available to diffuse into and block the nerve. There may also be increased local vascularity that increases removal of drug from the site.

INDIVIDUAL DRUG PROPERTIES (Table 14.1)

COCAINE

Cocaine is derived from the leaves of the *Erythroxylon coca* plant. It is used for topical anaesthesia and local vasoconstriction. Moffett's solution, which contains cocaine, adrenaline and sodium bicarbonate, has been used in the nasal cavities.

Table 14.1 Comparative pharmacology of local anaesthetics

Drug	Potency	Onset	Duration of action	pKa	Relative Lipid Solubility	% Protein Bound	Dose
Lignocaine	2	Fast	Medium	7.9	150	70	3–7 mg/kg*
Bupivacaine	8	Medium	Long	8.1	1,000	95	2 mg/kg
Levobupivacaine		Medium	Long				2 mg/kg
Ropivacaine	6	Medium	Long	8.1	300	94	2 mg/kg
Prilocaine	2	Fast	Medium	7.7	50	55	6–8 mg/kg*
Amethocaine	8	Slow	Long	8.5	200	75	

Note: *the dose of lignocaine is 3 mg/kg without adrenaline and 7 mg/kg with adrenaline
The dose of prilocaine is 6 mg/kg without adrenaline and 8 mg/kg with adrenaline

AMETHOCAINE

Amethocaine is an ester local anaesthetic. It is used in eye lens surgery as the sole anaesthetic agent. It is hydrolysed very slowly and is relatively toxic. It has a slow onset time and prolonged duration of action (4–6 hours). In the UK its use is restricted to topical anaesthesia (4%) cream (Ametop).

LIGNOCAINE

The most commonly used agent for local anaesthesia. It can be used for intravenous regional anaesthesia, peripheral nerve blocks, infiltration (0.5–1%), subarachnoid anaesthesia (5%), epidural anaesthesia (1–2%) and as a topical solution (2–4%) for anaesthesia of mucous membranes. It is also available as a 2% gel and as a 5% ointment. It is metabolised in the liver by dealkylation and excreted in the urine. The maximum safe dose of lignocaine is 3 mg/kg without adrenaline and 7 mg/kg with adrenaline (1:200000).

PRILOCAINE

This drug is frequently used for infiltration and intravenous regional anaesthesia. It is longer acting and less toxic. It is metabolised to *o*-toluidine, which converts haemoglobin to methaemoglobin, thus causing methaemoglobinaemia that is dose related (more likely when the prilocaine dose exceeds 600 mg). The treatment of this is ascorbic acid or methylene blue (1 mg/kg), which act as reducing agents. It is a component of Eutectic Mixture of Local Anaesthetic (EMLA).

BUPIVACAINE

May be used in a plain solution (0.25% and 0.5% with or without 1:200000 adrenaline), or in a hyperbaric solution (0.5%) containing 80 mg/ml glucose.

Its onset of action is slower than lignocaine. It has a longer duration of action reducing the need for repeated doses. It has a more toxic effect on the myocardium in overdosage than other local anaesthetic agents. It is highly protein bound and is metabolised in the liver. Bupivacaine is used for infiltration, peripheral nerve blockade, subarachnoid and extradural anaesthesia because of its prolonged duration of action. The maximum safe dose of bupivicaine is 2 mg/kg.

LEVOBUPIVACAINE

An isomer of bupivacaine. It is available as 0.25%, 0.5% and 0.75% solution. It is used in a similar manner to bupivacaine. The dose required to produce myocardial depression is higher for levobupivacaine compared with bupivacaine. Convulsions only occur at higher doses with levobupivacaine. The uses and dose of levobupivacaine are similar to bupivacaine.

ROPIVACAINE

An isomer of bupivacaine. Its local anaesthetic activity is similar to bupivacaine. It is metabolised in the liver.

Its main differences from bupivacaine are:

- it has a longer duration of action;
- it has decreased risk of cardiotoxicity;
- its differential sensory and motor blockade. Initially, due to its lower lipid solubility, there is reduced penetration of the large myelinated motor fibres. However, they will eventually get blocked after continuous infusion. Therefore, the motor blockade produced is slower in onset, less dense and of shorter duration than with bupivacaine.

EUTECTIC MIXTURE OF LOCAL ANAESTHETIC (EMLA)

Eutectic mixture is a mixture of local anaesthetics that melt to form oil at temperatures greater than 16°C. EMLA contains equal proportions (2.5%) of lignocaine and prilocaine. The mixture, being oil at room temperature, has a lower melting point.

It is used to provide surface analgesia before vascular cannulation or certain minor operations. It is applied to intact skin under an occlusive dressing for at least 45–60 minutes.

EMLA is avoided in patients with methaemoglobinaemia, infants less than 12 months of age and patients who are receiving treatment with methaemoglobin-inducing drugs.

EMLA should not be used on mucous membranes because it is rapidly absorbed systemically.

ADVERSE SIDE EFFECTS

ALLERGIC REACTIONS

Allergic reactions to the commonly used amide local anaesthetics are very rare. The main causes of allergic reactions are metabolites of esters such as para-aminobenzoic acid and preservatives such as methylparaben that are present in both esters and amides.

A patient reporting an allergy to a local anaesthetic must be taken seriously but a clear history will often reveal, for example, a vaso-vagal reaction during a dental procedure and not a true allergic reaction.

SYSTEMIC TOXICITY

The most common cause is accidental direct intravascular injection causing a rapid rise in plasma levels. Also, inadvertently exceeding the maximum safe dose of the local anaesthetic can lead to excess plasma concentrations and cause systemic toxicity.

There are other factors that can influence plasma concentration and hence toxicity caused by local anaesthetics.

Vascularity

The higher the blood flow, the more rapid is the increase in plasma concentration, for example, the intercostal space is extremely vascular and local anaesthetics deposited here will cause a more rapid rise in plasma levels than in the epidural space. Luckily for the surgical practitioner, absorption is slowest after skin infiltration anaesthesia. It follows that any vasoconstrictor containing solutions, by reducing local blood flow, will reduce absorption and slow the rise in plasma levels.

Patient factors

Patients who are elderly, debilitated or who have hepatic or renal dysfunction will be more likely to suffer from symptoms of toxicity with lower doses of local anaesthetics.

Pregnancy

Local anaesthetics cross the placenta readily but their effects are minimal.

MANIFESTATIONS OF SYSTEMIC TOXICITY

Adverse effects on the heart and brain occur because of the membrane stabilising effect of the local anaesthetics. The symptoms will depend upon the rate of increase in plasma concentration of the drug. An accidental intravenous overdose will lead to rapid cardio-respiratory collapse and central nervous system shutdown whereas a subcutaneous overdose will lead to a more gradual onset of symptoms giving a warning to stop giving the drug as soon as any symptoms develop.

Central nervous system

- Peri-oral tingling and numbness of the tongue
- Light-headed, drowsy, slurred speech
- Convulsions and coma.

Cardiovascular

- Myocardial depression leading to reduced cardiac output and a reduced systemic vascular resistance leading to hypotension
- Arrhythmias.

Respiratory

- Apnoea.

PREVENTING TOXICITY

Avoidance of accidental intravenous injection is the most important factor in preventing toxicity. Repeated aspiration is important especially if a large volume is being deposited in one site without movement of the needle. When adrenaline-containing solutions are being used an inadvertent intravenous injection will manifest itself after only a few millilitres of the drug by the development of a tachycardia. The patient should be monitored closely for early signs of toxicity.

TREATMENT OF TOXICITY

Facilities for treatment of local anaesthetic toxicity must always be available. The principles of cardiopulmonary resuscitation such as airway, breathing and circulation (ABC) must be followed in the event of an overdose causing a cardio-respiratory collapse.

The same principles apply for the treatment of convulsions and they must be stopped as quickly as possible using benzodiazepines or barbiturates.

Every person who performs any type of surgery must have the knowledge to be able to perform life support in case of a cardio-respiratory collapse. To this end, it should be a requirement that all practitioners keep up to date with resuscitation techniques by attending advanced life-support training classes.

CONTRAINDICATIONS TO LOCAL ANAESTHETICS

A true allergy or non-consent from the patient are the only absolute contra-indications to local anaesthesia. Relative contraindications include presence of infection and a coagulopathy.

INFECTION

Apart from the slight chance of spreading any infection, the main problem with applying local anaesthetics to infected tissue is that they may not work very well (see above). However, it may still be possible to perform an incision and drainage of an abscess under local anaesthesia.

COAGULOPATHY

This probably applies more for regional anaesthesia such as an epidural block. For superficial surgery, if the coagulation abnormality is not severe enough to prevent surgery, then local anaesthesia can almost certainly be performed.

USE OF LOCAL ANAESTHETICS

There are several ways that local anaesthetics can be used.

- Analgesia – to provide postoperative pain relief by wound infiltration.
- Regional anaesthesia such as epidurals or spinals.
- Topical anaesthesia to mucous membranes.
- Cutaneous anaesthesia, eg EMLA cream or Ametop.
- Local infiltration for excision of small tumours or suturing wounds.
- Peripheral nerve blocks, eg ulnar nerve.
- Intravenous regional anaesthesia (Bier's block).

There are two areas that probably merit a special mention.

- Scalp anaesthesia – the scalp has a nerve supply above and below an aponeurotic layer and therefore needs local anaesthetic deposited on either side of this layer. Also, being a very vascular area, adrenaline-containing solutions should be used.
- Digital nerve block – there are 4 nerve branches, 2 dorsal and 2 palmar. To perform this block infiltrate 1.0 ml around both nerves on each side of the digit, avoid too great a volume, and remember not to use vasopressors.

PRACTICAL ASPECTS

- A thorough preoperative assessment must always be performed.
- Check the drugs and resuscitation equipment.

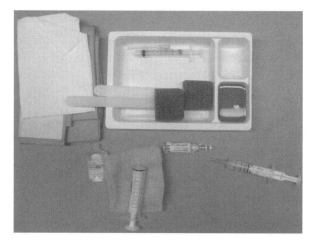

Figure 14.2 Pre-prepared pack.

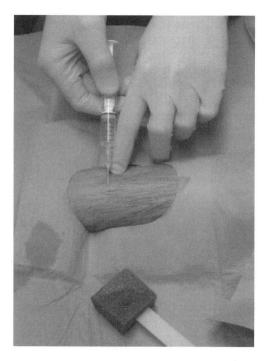

Figure 14.3 Infiltrating local anaesthetic after preparing surgical site.

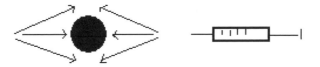

Figure 14.4 Fan infiltration – small lesion.

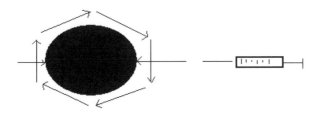

Figure 14.5 Encircling infiltration – large lesion.

- Keep within the maximum dose of the local anaesthetic by calculating the maximum volume that can be used before beginning the procedure. To do this remember that 1% solution = 10 mg/ml. For example, the maximum safe volume of lignocaine with adrenaline in a 100 kg person = *140 ml* as opposed to *18 ml* of 1% plain lignocaine in a 60 kg person. This illustration shows how the 'safe' volumes can vary widely.
- Clean the area to be operated upon with an antiseptic solution. Special packs may be prepared for this (Figure 14.2).
- Infiltrate the area using the predetermined dose of local anaesthetic. Local anaesthetic can be applied before skin preparation but it is probably best to perform the anaesthesia after prepping and draping (Figure 14.3). The patient should be warned that there may be a stinging sensation at first but this is very short lived. For the initial injection the use of fine needles, such as 23 G or 25 G, may lessen the initial pain on injection.
- For smaller lesions the local anaesthetic can be infiltrated in a 'fan' shaped pattern with only two puncture sites (Figure 14.4).
- For larger lesions this is not possible unless very long needles are used, which, apart from not being very practical, would also cause your patient some anxiety! Instead, the 'encircling' technique should be used whereby the needle is entered several times in order to infiltrate the anaesthetic all around the lesion (Figure 14.5).
- Wait for the local anaesthetic to work. This usually takes a couple of minutes.
- Test if the area is anaesthetised using the tip of a blade or needle.
- Proceed with the operation. Be prepared to infiltrate more anaesthetic into the wound during the operation if you need to.

POSTOPERATIVE CARE

Remember to prescribe analgesia such as paracetamol, codeine or NSAIDS. The patient should be advised to take some analgesia before the local wears off completely. The patient should not need more powerful analgesics, as the pain is usually mild to moderate only.

REFERENCES

Aitkenhead AR, Rowbotham D and Smith G (2001) *Textbook of Anaesthesia* 4th edn. Edinburgh: Churchill Livingstone.
Stoelting RK (2006) *Pharmacology and Physiology in Anesthetic Practice* 3rd edn. Philadelphia: Lippincott.
Calvey TN and Williams NE (2001) *Principles and Practices of Pharmacology for Anaesthetists* 4th edn. Oxford: Blackwell.
Yentis SM, Hirsch NP and Smith GB (2003) *Anaesthesia and Intensive Care A to Z: An Encyclopaedia of Principles and Practice* 3rd edn. Oxford: Butterworth Heinemann.

15 Operative Techniques for Minor Surgical Procedures

RAJESH AGGARWAL

INTRODUCTION

The aim of every operation is to ensure that the patient undergoes a procedure with the minimum of discomfort, and achieves a satisfactory end result. In the case of minor surgery, patients want to have the lesion removed in a painless manner, and end up with as neat a scar as possible. Indeed many patients are surprised that there will be a scar at all, and this must be explained in the first consultation. By following some simple rules regarding elective minor surgical procedures, it is possible to achieve a good result for many of our patients, with an almost invisible scar.

This entails adequate knowledge and the practical experience of the operating surgeon, in terms of planning the procedure, surgical technique, mode of excision, knowledge of instruments, sutures and other materials, and proficiency in the technical aspects of the procedure such as dissection and knot-tying.

PLANNING FOR THE PROCEDURE

When a patient attends a minor surgery clinic it is first necessary to make the diagnosis and confirm with the patient that they wish to have the lesion removed. However, prior to obtaining consent from the patient regarding the planned procedure, it is a pre-requisite that the operator is also comfortable to proceed. This involves consideration of the patient, the lesion and the facilities available in case of complication.

THE PATIENT

The majority of patients who attend for minor surgery are freely ambulatory, and generally well in themselves. However, patients may be on a drug which can affect the end result (Table 15.1), and should also be asked about any

Minor Surgical Procedures for Nurses and Allied Healthcare Professionals. Edited by Shirley Martin.
© 2007 John Wiley & Sons Limited

Table 15.1 Drugs to note in patients attending for minor surgical procedures

Drug	Effect
Anticoagulants, eg aspirin, warfarin	Excessive bleeding and postoperative haematoma formation
Immunosuppressive drugs, steroids	Poor wound healing

allergies, for example, to latex, local anaesthetics or any type of antiseptic fluid which may be used.

The patient's reason for requesting removal is also important. It may be because someone they know had skin cancer and they are anxious about the lesion. More frequently though, patients request removal for cosmetic reasons, and it is important in this instance to ensure the patient is aware of the end result, and also of any complications which may arise. Some patients also attend minor surgery clinics because they want a professional opinion on a skin lesion, rather than removal, and if it is not sinister they may not wish to have it excised.

THE LESION

Prior to commencement of any surgical procedure, the operator must ensure they are proficient to perform the task. For minor surgical procedure, a thorough knowledge of surface anatomy can help to ensure that the unexpected does not occur, such as puncture of an artery or cutting of a nerve. For very large lesions, removal may not be possible due to the maximal doses of local anaesthetic that can be used. Similarly, some small lesions such as ganglions necessitate the use of a tourniquet which can only be tolerated under general anaesthetic. If there is any uncertainty regarding removal of a skin lesion, it is appropriate to obtain senior advice, or ask the patient to return for another appointment.

When planning removal of the lesion, it is also necessary to ensure the lesion and its surrounding areas are clean, dry and free of any hair. If the lesion is over hairy skin, it is best shaved with a sterile razor. However, lesions on the hairy scalp may be exposed with the use of K-Y jelly, rather than leaving the patient with an unsightly bald patch.

THE FACILITIES AVAILABLE

As mentioned above, if the operator is not confident in removing a lesion, it is best left alone for senior review. With the introduction of minor surgery clinics in the community, and procedures sometimes being carried out in the evenings there may be a lack of specialist back-up should things go seriously wrong. This is extremely unlikely, but it is important to plan ahead and if there is a suspicion that the lesion is very deep, very large, or abutting some major structures, it is best referred for assessment by a more experienced member of the team.

SURGICAL TECHNIQUES

Each minor surgical procedure can be divided into five stages: skin incision, dissection and exposure, removal, haemostasis, and skin closure. Haemostasis and anaesthetic considerations have been considered elsewhere in this book, and will not be discussed further here.

SKIN INCISION

Deciding where to make the incision depends upon its location on the body, its shape, and the presumed diagnosis of the lesion. In 1861, Langer described lines across the body which would result in optimal healing and the neatest scars (Chapter 13, Figure 13.2). These are now known as Langer's lines and should be borne in mind when planning an elective incision. As a rule of thumb, it is best to make incisions in natural wrinkle lines which can be located by asking the patient to contract the underlying muscles.

The majority of lesions on the skin are spherical or ellipsoid in shape, and if attached to the skin, an elliptical incision should be made. It is of course essential to remove the entire lesion, with a 3–4 mm margin of normal skin around it. Incising in an elliptical manner may lead to a longer scar, but the end result will be superior to a circular incision once closed. Due to the excess tension of a circular incision, it is almost certain to lead to the formation of a 'dog-ear' at one end of the scar.

However, if the lesion is underlying the skin, ie has normal skin overlying it, then it is not always necessary to make an elliptical incision and a transverse incision across the widest part of the lump can suffice. The commonest example of this is when excising a lipoma. Once the incision is made, the scar is undermined on both sides, enabling fairly large lesions to be removed with relatively small scars.

It is also important to ensure when making the incision that the scalpel blade is at right angles to the skin, rather than at an oblique angle. An oblique incision will lead to a broad scar when the incision is brought back together, whereas a vertical incision will produce a narrow, linear scar. When the skin is incised, it is also helpful to use the thumb and forefinger of the non-dominant hand to place the skin under tension. Deciding upon the length and shape of the incision at the outset will also produce a better scar than if the lesion has to be lengthened. This can be aided by use of a sterile marker pen at the outset, providing a line to cut along. Finally, the incision should be made with one stroke, rather than numerous small incisions which traumatise the skin to a greater extent, leading to a more vigorous inflammatory response and hence a poorer end result.

DISSECTION AND EXPOSURE

Once the initial incision has been made it is necessary to dissect out the offending lesion. The techniques used can be divided into sharp or blunt dissection. Sharp dissection is either with a scalpel blade, or the blades of a pair of scissors, with the aim being to cut through tissue planes. This method is highly effective and produces the least amount of tissue trauma, though it can lead to inadvertent injury of adjacent tissues and structures. Diathermy may also be used as a form of sharp dissection, in the same manner as a scalpel blade.

Blunt dissection is performed by placing closed scissors or retracting forceps into the wound, and opening the blades. Hence the blunt end of the instrument pushes the tissues apart, and will often reveal rather than cut through vessels and nerves. This process is more time consuming, though it can be a safer method. Blunt dissection can also be carried out by the operator's fingers placed into the wound, or even by spreading the wound retractors apart.

Retraction during any surgical procedure is almost more important than dissection. This is because it is only with good retraction and subsequent exposure that the appropriate tissues to dissect come into view. Retraction can be hand-held with 'skin hooks', 'cat's paw', or Langenbeck non-traumatic retractors, though this entails the use of an assistant. Self retracting forceps are useful for larger incisions but, because of their size, can get in the way for smaller incisions. If attempting to dissect the posterior aspect of a skin lump, a good view may be attained by grasping the lump itself with tissue-holding Alliss forceps, and using these to retract the lump laterally. It should also be stated as a general rule that if one is using traumatic instruments to retract with such as tissue grasping forceps, it is advisable to only take hold of the tissue which will be removed at the end of the procedure. This is to avoid unnecessary harm to the remaining tissue, which can augment the tissue inflammatory response.

REMOVAL

Once the lump has been dissected from the surrounding tissues, it is not simply a matter of removing it and placing it in the histology pot. The operator must ensure that the lesion has been removed in its entirety. This can be particularly difficult when removing a lipoma, especially if it is adherent to the surrounding tissues. Incomplete removal will lead to recurrence. In the case of sebaceous cysts, it is advisable, though not mandatory, to remove the lump without breaching the capsule and subsequent leak of the cyst contents.

This is because leakage can lead to an increased of risk postoperative wound infection.

The simplest method to reduce risk of recurrence or wound infection is to ensure the cavity is clean and devoid of any pathological tissue. It may be advisable to rinse with sterile antiseptic solution if there has been a leakage of cyst contents.

SKIN CLOSURE

If two skin edges are brought together in the absence of tension, any wound should heal within a period of seven to ten days. However, the mode of closure is important, to achieve that 'almost invisible' scar. Firstly, if the dissection and removal has left a large cavity, usually only for a lipoma, it is necessary to place some stitches across the cavity to prevent subsequent seroma or haematoma formation. The stitches should be placed across the wound, in an interrupted fashion, using absorbable suture material. This will also help to reduce the tension on the skin sutures.

Bleeding from the wound is most likely to be from the fine capillaries, and will stop spontaneously, or once the skin edges are brought together, due to the effect of tamponade. Brisk bleeding from a visible blood vessel can be controlled with pressure, and again will stop once the wound edges are brought together. If it is within the cavity of the lesion which has been removed, it may be managed by diathermy of the vessel, or the placement of a subcutaneous stitch.

Closure of the skin can be performed through use of sutures, sterile strips, skin clips or adhesive glues. These materials will be explained in a later section; the overall aim is to bring the skin edges together with the minimal amount of tissue trauma, and wound tension. In terms of wound tension, especially if a wide ellipse has been made, it can be beneficial to undermine the wound edges away from the subcutaneous fat. This provides more laxity to the wound edges, resulting in a better end result.

Once skin closure has been completed, it is important to inform the patient of whether suture removal is necessary, and also to apply a suitable dressing to the wound. Dressings are useful to protect the wound from contamination, absorb any secretions, provide some additional support during the healing phase and to limit excessive movements during the healing phase. Standard practice is to apply a non-adherent dressing such as Mepore Pro which will not disrupt the wound when removed. The patient is advised to keep the skin over and around the wound clean and dry for the first 48 hours, and then to change dressings only if necessary. Suture removal is anticipated at 4–5 days for wounds on the face, 10 days on the back and approximately 7 days everywhere else on the body. This is because of the differences in the blood supply and skin thickness of the different parts of the body, the face possessing the thinnest skin and most concentrated blood supply.

INSTRUMENTATION

During minor surgical procedures the operator is confronted with a 'minor surgery' set of between 10 and 20 instruments for use during an operation. In fact, it is not really necessary to use all these instruments and a basic set consisting of just six instruments can suffice for the majority of procedures (Table 15.2). The remainder of the instruments are variations upon this theme, ie fine needle holders, fine toothed forceps, tissue-holding forceps, etc.

Additional instruments are used for retraction and have been discussed in the previous section.

MATERIALS FOR SKIN CLOSURE

As mentioned above, skin closure simply necessitates the apposition of the two skin edges for a short period of time. The wide array of suture materials available can be daunting, though most practitioners restrict themselves to their personal selection of preferred materials. The most convenient method of defining suture materials is to divide them into three broad categories: absorbable vs. non-absorbable; synthetic vs. natural; and braided vs. monofilament (Table 15.3).

Table 15.2 Instruments required for minor surgery (the bare essentials)

Instrument	Uses
Scalpel plus blade	Incision, sharp dissection
Pair of toothed dissecting forceps	Retraction and exposure; skin closure
Pair of mosquito forceps	Blunt dissection
Needle holder	Skin closure
Straight stitch scissors	Cutting sutures
Curved MacIndoe scissors	Sharp and blunt dissection

Table 15.3 A classification of suture materials

Absorbable	Synthetic	Braided	Coated polygactin (Vicryl)
		Monofilament	Monocryl monofilament suture
	Natural	Braided	Plain catgut
		Monofilament	–
Non-absorbable	Synthetic	Braided	Nylon
		Monofilament	Monofilament propylene (Prolene)
	Natural	Braided	Braided silk (Mersilk)
		Monofilament	–

Generally, it is advisable to use the suture that causes the minimal tissue reaction. The most popular types used in minor surgical practice are monofilament, synthetic sutures such as Prolene, or Monocryl. The monofilament nature leads to a reduced tissue reaction and also diminishes the risk of wound infection. The best end result is achieved by use of interrupted, nonabsorbable sutures which are removed at a suitable time interval. A subcuticular stitch using an absorbable monofilament suture (e.g. Monocryl) also provides a neat scar, and takes less time to insert than interrupted sutures. However, to attain sufficient strength in the wound, the incision needs to be longer than 5 cm. Continuous stitches over the wound are not useful in minor surgery as they do not achieve adequate tension in small scars, and are difficult to remove. The benefit of using braided or multi-filament sutures is that they are easier to tie due to the locking effect of the suture material.

Skin closure clips are not generally used for minor surgical procedures, though they enable a wound to be quickly and accurately closed, and provide good skin apposition. However, they necessitate a special instrument for removal, and may be uncomfortable for the patient.

Sterile strips for wound closure are used as an alternative or a supplement to skin closure with sutures. They must be applied on to a dry and clean wound, and good apposition can be achieved for fairly small incisions. They have the benefit of ease of removal; the patient can just soak in the bath after a few days and the strips will simply lift off. Furthermore, the patient does not have to make a further appointment for removal.

Tissue adhesives can be used for the closure of minor skin wounds without suturing, and work by polymerisation upon contact with water. Histoacryl blue (enbucrilate) is the most common type used, applied evenly along the skin edges and held in position for one minute. Anything that comes into contact with Histoacryl will adhere to it, so the operating practitioner must be particularly aware of their clothes, gloves, fingers and swabs when applying the adhesive. Tissue adhesive is commonly used in the Emergency Department for closure of scalp wounds, and on young children when local anaesthetic is unnecessary. As with sterile strips, this also eliminates the need for a follow-up consultation.

STITCHING AND KNOT-TYING

It is beyond the scope of a textbook to train someone how to effectively tie knots during minor surgical practice. This must be learnt on synthetic models which are widely available for knot-tying, suture practice and skin lesion excision. However, there are a few principles which must be adhered to in order to achieve the optimal end result.

Suturing may be divided into three types: simple interrupted, vertical mattress interrupted, or subcuticular continuous. Simple interrupted sutures are commonly laid with a curved needle which should be inserted through the skin at right angles, and the exit-tract should also be at right angles. This is achieved by gliding the needle through the tissue with a supination movement of the wrist, rather than by forcing or pushing the needle through. The sutures should be placed symmetric distances from the wound edges, and uniform distances apart. For an elliptical wound, it is advisable to place one stitch at one end of the incision, and the next stitch on the opposite end. Gradually, the stitches are placed closer toward the middle of the incision; this can result in tension-free closure, and prevent the formation of dog ears at the edges. Simple interrupted sutures are the optimal method of wound closure. However, if the wound is difficult to close, vertical mattress sutures may be a suitable alternative. With this type of closure the skin edges are opposed at a subcutaneous and subcuticular level, strengthening their apposition.

Finally, subcuticular stitches are useful when there is minimal risk of subcutaneous haematoma formation. The stitch begins at one end of the wound and passes backwards and forwards, under the surface of the skin, until the opposite wound edge has been reached. This type of closure leaves a good end result, and is used when the wound edges can be brought together closely without tension.

Knot-tying is something which develops with practice, whether it is on the back of a chair, or in the surgical skills laboratory. The two types of knots commonly used in all types of surgery are the 'hand-tie' and the 'instrument-tie'. Hand-tied knots are more difficult to learn, and use more suture material. In minor surgery, it is commonplace to instrument-tie as this uses less suture material and is an easier skill to acquire. When laying the first knot, it is important to ensure that the skin edges are everted as this will lead to a better end result.

SUMMARY

Minor surgical procedures, irrespective of their name, can be quite daunting and have the propensity to lead to major complications when practised by inexperienced operators. The skills necessary to deliver a satisfactory end result to the patient are not complex, and can be learnt over a short period of time. However, as with any surgical procedure, it is important to follow simple principles as set out in this chapter. Proficiency will only develop with repeated exposure and practice, and this chapter should only be viewed as a guide to operative practice.

16 Haemostasis and Cautery for Minor Procedures

PARVINDERPAL SAINS

SECURING HAEMOSTASIS

Haemostasis can be defined as 'halting the flow of blood'. The body's own clotting mechanisms do of course play an important role in securing haemostasis as a result of trauma. However, minimising blood loss is part of good surgical technique and safe medical practice. Meticulous haemostasis at all stages of operative procedures is vital to good outcomes by reducing the risk of wound haematomas, infection and dehiscence. In the worst case scenarios bleeding from minor operation sites can lead to significant blood loss and is distressing for the patient.

Bleeding will occur after a minor procedure such as a skin ellipse excision. This will arise from vessels that have been cut in the subcutis and along the dermal wound edge. The bleeding may be a slow ooze from minute capillaries or more rapid from a few larger vessels. The vessels are seldom of large calibre but even moderate bleeding should be controlled prior to closure. The development of haematomas and persistent bleeding after discharge will be prevented by a meticulous approach to haemostasis.

Initial haemostasis in any surgical circumstance is achieved by pressure over the bleeding point with a finger and gauze. This method is very effective, especially for venous bleeds, and it is surprising how much haemostasis can be achieved.

Larger vessels can be tied off by the use of ligatures or electro-cautery, which will be discussed in more detail below. Once adequate haemostasis has been achieved, closure of the wound can be performed which in itself will promote haemostasis by apposition of the skin edges. This provides pressure at the wound edges and also significant haemostasis through blood clotting mechanisms, which is the first stage of wound healing. If any doubt remains postoperatively, then a pressure dressing consisting of gauze and a second adhesive dressing can be applied over the dressing covering the wound.

Minor Surgical Procedures for Nurses and Allied Healthcare Professionals. Edited by Shirley Martin.
© 2007 John Wiley & Sons Limited

LIGATURES

Large vessels that can be seen bleeding in the wound can be ligated by the use of a haemostat and ligature. The vessel is grasped with the haemostat and a fine ligature is applied below the haemostat. Once a knot has been secured the haemostat is removed and the ligature ends are cut short.

The material used for ligatures is the same as that used for sutures. When selecting a ligature the following factors have to be considered:

- whether the material is to be absorbed;
- what thickness (gauge or calibre) is to be used;
- the likely intensity of the body's reaction.

For the purposes of minor surgery, absorbable sutures are normally used. The absorption rate varies greatly. The most commonly used is polyglactin 910 (coated Vicryl) with a gauge of 3.0 or 4.0. This is a synthetic, braided (multifilament) ligature which handles and knots easily and is more flexible than monofilament ligatures. It is fully absorbed within ninety days with the 'rapide' version being absorbed within ten days. The tensile strength provided is adequate for the purposes of minor surgical procedures. If the ligature is to be applied close to the skin surface it is advisable to use an undyed version so as not to tattoo the skin.

ELECTROCAUTERY

Electrocautery or surgical diathermy has been used in operating theatres for over a century. It involves the passage of a high frequency alternating current (AC) through the body tissue from one electrode to another (active and return electrodes). At the point of local concentration of the current a temperature of up to 1000°C can be achieved. The AC in the United Kingdom is delivered at a frequency of approximately 50 Hz. The effect on tissue is dependent on the current. A current in the region of 80–100 mA will induce cardiac arrhythmia. However, an increase in the frequency of the current will reduce the neuromuscular response with abolishment at frequencies above 50 kHz. At this frequency currents up to 500 mA can be safely passed through the tissue. As the current passes though the patient it is impeded by the tissues creating heat within the tissues with a maximum point produced wherever the current is locally concentrated. Diathermy can be monopolar or bipolar.

Monopolar diathermy

These circuits are the most commonly used in larger surgical cases. High frequency current is provided by a generator diathermy machine (Figure 16.1)

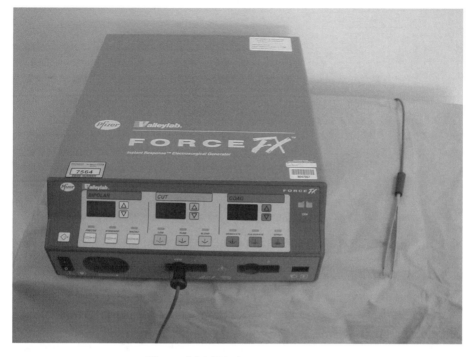

Figure 16.1 Diathermy generator.

to an active electrode held by a surgeon. The current density is maximal at
the tip of the electrode, which is in contact with tissue. Maximum heat is
generated at this point within the tissue. The current then dissipates throughout the body and is returned to the generator via a 'plate' electrode which is
placed on the patient. The plate electrode covers approximately 80 cm^2 so as
not to concentrate the current and cause burns. Monopolar diathermy is very
uncommon in the minor surgery setting.

Bipolar diathermy

In bipolar diathermy both the active and return electrodes are part of one
electrosurgical unit. This is usually in the form of a pair of forceps (Figure
16.2), negating the need for a plate to be placed on the patient. One tine of
the forceps carries current to the tissue (active electrode) and the second tine
returns it to the generator (return electrode). The current traverses the tissue
between the two tines. Therefore, the grasped tissue will be heated. Low
power current can be used in bipolar electrocautery as only a small amount
of tissue is exposed. This makes it ideal for use in minor surgical procedures
and is an inherently safer system.

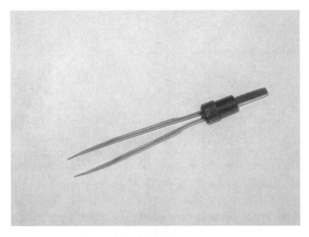

Figure 16.2 Bipolar diathermy forceps.

Safety and hazards

All equipment used should meet the required safety standards and regular maintenance should be carried out. All personnel using the equipment need to be adequately trained in its use and a user manual should be made available at all times.

Thermoelectric burns are the main danger from electrocautery and are always accidental rather than caused by faulty equipment. Common mistakes include touching the side of the wound with unprotected forceps, activating the current at the wrong time, applying current to the wrong area or using too much power.

A significant error to make when using bipolar diathermy is assuming that insulation that covers the majority of the tines is fully intact. It is a common finding that the insulation has broken down, potentially allowing a pathway for current to pass into tissue other than the target tissue. The control pedal for operating the diathermy should be under the control of the operating surgeon only in order to minimise the risk of activating the machine at the wrong time. The power dial settings should be checked by the surgeon before activation. The forceps should be returned to a quiver when not in use. Another important consideration is to use a spirit based skin preparation which should be allowed to evaporate prior to activation of the diathermy as this may ignite it.

In summary, electrocautery can be used to close vessels. Damage to adjacent non-bleeding tissue should be minimised during the procedure. Grasping the bleeding vessel with bipolar forceps permits precise targeting for coagulation. The area at the cauterised site must be dry for the device to work optimally, and this dry field may be maintained by applying gauze. In general, electrocautery should be sufficient but not excessive. Not every pinpoint bleeder needs to be treated, and the wound edge should be treated sparingly if at all. Overuse of the cautery device can devitalise tissue at the closure site, impeding healing and creating a reservoir of necrotic tissue that is vulnerable to infection.

17 Future Prospects

SHIRLEY MARTIN

At the beginning of this book it was shown how new opportunities have arisen for enthusiastic healthcare practitioners to take on diverse roles, which is a key event in the delivery of patient care. These can be challenging and fulfilling, and during the transitional process practitioners can encounter both positive and negative attitudes in others.

Government proposals and public attitudes are changing towards patient care, which is more than ever expected to be prompt, resourceful and efficient. As a result there are continuous changes in medical training and career paths and surgical teams have often been under pressure, with the result that junior doctors fear the loss of training opportunities and surgical experience.

Surgical care practitioners are currently at the forefront of many discussions, including their working title, curriculum, scope of practice, regulation and clinical supervision. Some doctors have openly objected that surgical care practitioners have a detrimental effect on doctors' surgical training. In addition many of them maintain that nurses and non-medically qualified professionals have little training and have not attained full medical qualifications so should not be allowed to 'wield' a scalpel in order to reduce waiting lists. This resistance to change is inevitable. Further negative constraints have emerged with the announcement that many large NHS Trusts have run up huge deficits. This has sometimes led to a reduction in training budgets and in the number of the most highly specialised (and hence most expensive) nurses, many of whom have been forced to focus on more general health work. Many specialist nurses have been asked to work shifts on wards related to their speciality or appropriately, in operating theatres, work normally carried out by agency and bank staff. It's been reported that some specialised nurses have been targeted for redundancy (Harrison 2006). This has led to a disruption of practitioner led clinics, with patient enquiries not immediately dealt with.

Unpublished reports higlighted that one specific Trust undertook a peer review of each nurse specialist which comprised small audit teams. The team, headed by the Head of Nursing Lead Nurse and representatives from the directorate, involved observation of Clinical Nurse Specialists in practice,

Minor Surgical Procedures for Nurses and Allied Healthcare Professionals. Edited by Shirley Martin.
© 2007 John Wiley & Sons Limited

shadowing them, reviewing nurse-led clinics, their discussions with personnel and interactions with consultants and medical colleagues.

Downgrading higher band specialist nurses and surgical care practitioners under Agenda for Change has also been widely reported as Trusts have been unable to pay them at a higher rate. In some cases it has been noted that consultants have been so angry at this that they have sought advice from lawyers, and have even offered to give up part of their salary to prevent nurse practitioners leaving.

On a positive note, successful practitioners will have trained in a wide range of client care, and the scope of their role has expanded to include system management and professional role development. Examples include the admission process of clerking and preparing patients for surgery, performing hernia repairs, varicose vein surgery, cystoscopy/hysteroscopy and minor lid procedures, mostly without complications. For some there have been opportunities across a wide area of healthcare provision, including assessing emergency admissions and performing Accident and Emergency duties, providing night and on-call cover, and prescribing. Such attributes encourage assertiveness, autonomy and clear decision-making in dealing with clinical problems while interacting with primary and secondary care doctors.

However, particular care should be taken to avoid the role becoming task orientated only. For example, performing nothing but simple minor skin surgery (skin tags) or endoscopic procedures on a daily basis can become mundane and tedious.

This book has introduced non-medically qualified practitioners who often hold a wealth of experience, which can be beneficial to the surgical trainee. They can play a key part in training junior surgeons in basic surgical techniques and other outpatient procedures. Much emphasis must be based around the 'Team'. It is vital that acceptance, communication and understanding is relayed between all members of the team.

In conclusion, through the challenging evolution of non-medically qualified practitioner roles and by becoming more fully involved with the needs of patients the individual can achieve great job satisfaction. On this path it is essential that advanced practitioners do not become competitive or compare themselves with medical colleagues but evolve as unique practitioners in their own right providing appropriate services to meet changing healthcare needs. These are exciting times, with many new horizons opening. It is however clear that far reaching cultural changes within the medical profession are essential, accompanied by support from senior medical practitioners, if the potential benefits to patients are to be fully realised.

REFERENCES

Harrison S (2006) The tide has turned for specialists as Trusts try to balance their books. *Nursing Standard*. June 7, vol 20, No 39.

Glossary and Role Definitions

Associate specialist

A medically qualified practitioner trained in one of the nine surgical specialties, gynaecology or ophthalmology who may or may not be registered on the specialist register.

Clinical logbook

An electronic or hard copy record demonstrating completed clinical activities and practical expertise.

Clinical nurse specialist

A registered nurse specialised in medical or surgical clinical practice.

Clinical supervisor

An accredited consultant surgeon, with the responsibility for a trainee within, for example, a surgical team.

Competence and competencies

Competence – the aptitude of a professional conducting their practice, which requires the use of professional judgment.
Competencies – the specific skills taught and tested in an educational process.

Consultant surgeon

A medically qualified practitioner trained in one of the nine specialties of surgery, gynaecology or ophthalmology who is responsible for treatment and care of patients in the theatre and surgical wards.

Minor Surgical Procedures for Nurses and Allied Healthcare Professionals. Edited by Shirley Martin.
© 2007 John Wiley & Sons Limited

Curriculum framework

An educational policy document providing the background, development, entry criteria, definitions, structure of education and training, and assessment strategy for trainees.

Educational profile

A document demonstrating aspects of academic achievements and theoretical and practical learning. It should also include formative and summative assessments and records of meetings.

Extended surgical team

The extended surgical team is made up of the traditional surgical team and other medically and non-medically qualified healthcare professionals who perform surgical procedures under supervision.

The extended surgical team is composed of:

- general practitioners with special interest in surgery;
- surgical care practitioners;
- surgical nurse practitioners;
- endoscopists;
- emergency care practitioners.

Foundation Year 1 and 2 doctor

A medically qualified practitioner's training in basic surgical techniques before embarking on training as a specialist in one of the specialties of medicine.

General practitioner

A general practitioner (GP) or family doctor is a physician who is responsible for treating acute and chronic illnesses in the primary care setting. Some also perform minor surgical procedures.

Perioperative specialist practitioner

The opposite role to the surgical care practitioner. It involves pre- and post-operative duties in the surgical setting but not performing intra-operative surgical interventions.

Personal profile

Individual documentation of current employment and previous development. It provides evidence of learning, supporting achievements of theoretical or clinical development. Professional written reflections on development will form a key part of the portfolio of evidence.

Portfolio of evidence

A professional portfolio demonstrating individual development, progression and achievements over a period of time. The portfolio should include a personal and educational profile including competencies, clinical logbook, and record of academic work.

Practitioner

This term encompasses all health professionals working with patients. Used when describing activities believed to be generic.

Surgical care practitioner (former title surgical assistant)

A non-medical practitioner working in clinical practice as a member of the extended surgical team, who performs surgical intervention, preoperative and postoperative care under the direction and supervision of a consultant surgeon. (2006, Department of Health). The Curriculum Framework for the Surgical Care Practitioner.

Index

Minor Surgical Procedures for Nurses and Allied Healthcare Professionals. Edited by Shirley Martin.
© 2007 John Wiley & Sons Limited